LEARNING RESOURCES CTR/NEW ENGLAND TECH.
GEN   RC641.5.K37 1988
Kass, Lawren   Pernicious anemia /

3 0147 0000 4881 2

RC641.5 .K37 1988

Kass

T5-CUL-024

Pernicious anemia

DATE

188
1989
2 6 199

This is an authorized facsimile, made from the master copy of the original book.

Out-of-Print Books on Demand is a publishing service of UMI. The program offers xerographic reprints of more than 100,000 books that are no longer in print.

The primary focus is academic and professional resource materials originally published by university presses, academic societies and trade book publishers worldwide.

U·M·I Out-of-Print Books on Demand

University Microfilms International
A Bell & Howell Information Company
300 N. Zeeb Road, Ann Arbor, Michigan 48106
800-521-0600 OR 313/761-4700

Printed in 1988 by xerographic process
on acid-free paper

LAWRENCE KASS, M.S., M.D.

Associate Professor of Internal Medicine
and Research Associate
The Thomas Henry Simpson Memorial Institute
for Medical Research
The University of Michigan
Ann Arbor, Michigan

PERNICIOUS ANEMIA

VOLUME

VII

IN THE SERIES

MAJOR PROBLEMS IN INTERNAL MEDICINE

Lloyd H. Smith, Jr., M.D., *Editor*

W. B. SAUNDERS COMPANY • PHILADELPHIA • LONDON • TORONTO • 1976

2019981

W. B. Saunders Company: West Washington Square
Philadelphia, PA 19105   .

12 Dyott Street
London, WC1A 1DB

833 Oxford Street
Toronto, Ontario M8Z 5T9, Canada

Library of Congress Cataloging in Publication Data

Kass, Lawrence.
  Pernicious anemia.

  (Major problems in internal medicine; v. 7)
  Bibliography: p.
  Includes index.
  1. Pernicious anemia. I. Title. [DNLM: 1. Anemia,
Pernicious. W1 MA492T v. 7 / WH165 K19p]
RC641.5.K37   616.1'52   75-8180
ISBN 0-7216-5295-6

Pernicious Anemia   ISBN 0-7216-5295-6

© 1976 by the W. B. Saunders Company. Copyright under the International Copyright
Union. All rights reserved. This book is protected by copyright. No part of it may
be reproduced, stored in a retrieval system, or transmitted in any form or by any means,
electronic, mechanical, photocopying, recording or otherwise, without written permission from the publisher. Made in the United States of America. Press of W. B. Saunders Company. Library of Congress catalogue card number 75-8180.

Last digit is the print number: 9   8   7   6   5   4   3   2   1

EDITOR'S FOREWORD

This is an auspicious year for a comprehensive monograph on pernicious anemia. Although previously described by Combe (1822) and Addison (1849), the disease received its English name exactly 100 years ago in an editorial entitled "Pernicious Anaemia: A new disease."[1] It was 50 years ago that Minot and Murphy announced the efficacy of liver therapy in this previously fatal disorder.[2] Therefore, it is most appropriate that Dr. William P. Murphy has personally written a foreword to this volume.

The clinical and pathological description of a disease and the discovery of a highly effective form of therapy might be thought to mark the close of a chapter in medical research. Quite the contrary, it stimulated a chain of basic and clinical research which still continues. The study of pernicious anemia is one of the best examples of the seminal role of clinical research in opening new areas of basic biological investigation. As documented in this book, the ramifications have extended into crystallography, organic chemistry, intermediary metabolism in man and bacteria, the physiology of transport, immunology, neurochemistry, genetics, cell biology, and cytology. The dietary requirement for cobalamins represents human "parasitism" on bacteria, since vitamin B_{12} is exclusively of microbiological origin. Elaborate mechanisms have evolved for the capture of the 1 microgram of this vitamin necessary for the maintenance of health, via intrinsic factor, highly specific transport in the ileum, and the transcobalamins. The vitamin is enzymatically converted into the forms required as cofactors for methionine synthesis or for propionic acid metabolism. Disorders have been described at virtually all steps in this sequence from the availability of the vitamin in the diet to its enzymatic activation to cofactor potential. As Dr. Kass has stated, "The story of pernicious anemia is one of the great dramas in the history of medicine." It is also a case history of the fertile interaction of clinical and biological research to the mutual benefit of medicine and biology.

No longer pernicious, deficiency of vitamin B_{12} still has its lessons to teach us. In this monograph, Dr. Kass has written a definitive summary of our knowledge concerning pernicious anemia. There is a rational progression from history to biochemistry in an interesting and well told story. It will be a point of departure for new chapters yet to be written.

LLOYD H. SMITH, JR., M.D.

---

1. Pernicious Anemia: A new disease. Med Times Gazette 2:581, 1876.
2. Minot G., Murphy W. P.: Treatment of pernicious anemia by a special diet. JAMA 87:470, 1926.

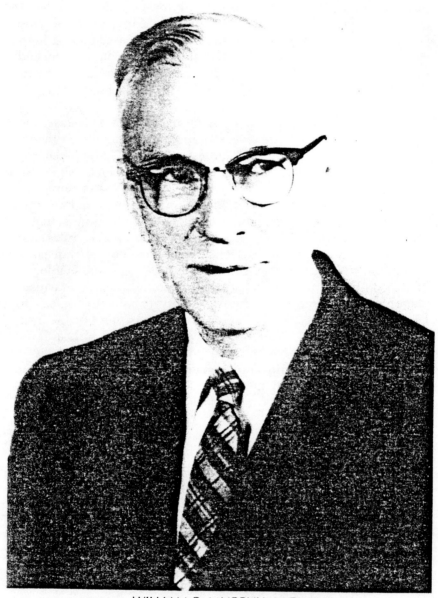

WILLIAM P. MURPHY, M.D.
Nobel Laureate in Physiology and Medicine 1934

FOREWORD

Following an internship and residency at the Peter Bent Brigham Hospital, Dr. Kass has had a brilliant career as a teacher and researcher in the field of hematology. He is presently working at the Thomas Henry Simpson Memorial Institute, which was founded in 1924 for research in hematology, with particular emphasis on pernicious anemia.

Perhaps Dr. Kass became interested in pernicious anemia while he was one of my students at the Peter Bent Brigham Hospital, for he concludes in his monograph that pernicious anemia is "one of the great dramas in the history of medicine." After a scholarly and interesting review of the early reports of "anemia" and efforts to treat the disease, finally designated as pernicious anemia, Dr. Kass comes to the conclusion that the effective remedy of pernicious anemia dated from the report of Drs. Minot and Murphy presented at the Meeting of the Association of American Physicians in May of 1926 and published in the *Journal of the American Medical Association* in August of the same year. This work, which included a series of forty-five cases, was started by me at the Peter Bent Brigham Hospital in the fall of 1924, the same year that saw the founding of the Thomas Henry Simpson Memorial Institute.

Dr. Kass has described my experience with my first pernicious anemia patient in the hospital. Following the successful treatment of this patient, there was little difficulty in getting the utmost cooperation from the hospital staff. However, the treatment was not always easy, for many of my patients had difficulty chewing and ingesting one-quarter to one-half pound of liver, which we had decided was the proper dose. Many patients were actually ill, and the liver was unfortunately not always served in the most appetizing manner despite the fact that I enjoyed the greatest rapport with the Dietetic Department and the nursing staff.

Because of this difficulty, we devised a method of grinding the liver into a fine pulp so that it could be drunk or even, in some rare instances, given by stomach tube. Then, because even the pulp was not too well received by some of the patients, I made a water soluble extract which could be taken more easily. This established the fact that the potent substance in liver was water soluble.

Later Dr. Edwin J. Cohn made a powder extract of this water soluble material, which in some ways simplified the treatment. This extract proved to be unpleasant to take and also expensive. Therefore, I later made an injectable solution from it. This was found to be irritating and somewhat painful when given by intramuscular injection. At this point Dr. Guy W. Clark of the Lederle Laboratories purified and concentrated this material so that 1 cc contained the effective substance found in a half pound of liver. This was the first commercial liver extract to be marketed. Today the effective substance in liver, which is vitamin B_{12}, is available in purified form so that it can be used in place of the original liver extract if so desired.

Dr. Kass's monograph on pernicious anemia not only is desirable reading for the younger generations of doctors who are interested in the subject, but it also provides a rich background of information for the many interested laymen.

William P. Murphy

PREFACE

The story of pernicious anemia is one of the great dramas in the history of medicine. From the opening scenes in which pernicious anemia was described by Combe in 1822 and Addison in 1849, to the "thickening of the plot" with the clinical accounts of Biermer in 1872 and the morphological observations of Ehrlich in 1880, to the *dénouement* in the great empirical discovery of liver therapy by Minot and Murphy in 1926, and the final scenes culminating in the isolation and crystallization of vitamin B_{12} from liver extracts by Rickes et al. and Smith in 1948, the elucidation of the molecular structure of vitamin B_{12} by Hodgkin in 1956, and the total synthesis of vitamin B_{12} by Woodward in 1972, the saga of pernicious anemia remains one of the most compelling accounts in man's conquest and understanding of disease.

Although historical, clinical, morphological, and biochemical aspects are covered in considerable detail, the main emphasis and purpose of this book is to attempt to place the pathophysiological and pathogenetic aspects of pernicious anemia into a contemporary perspective. This approach has been facilitated by the many recent advances in cytogenetics, cytochemistry, biochemistry, autoimmunity, and tissue culture studies that have advanced our knowledge of the pathogenesis of this disease.

This monograph on pernicious anemia was written in the golden anniversary year of the founding in 1924 of the Thomas Henry Simpson Memorial Institute for Medical Research, the only institute of hematology in the world, that was originally founded to discover a cure for pernicious anemia. Although the cure for pernicious anemia was discovered two years later in 1926, investigations are still being carried out at the Simpson Memorial Institute and the University of Michigan Medical Center relating to some of the original unanswered questions regarding the pathophysiology of pernicious anemia and the mystery of the megaloblastic lesion.

I thank Drs. Chris J. D. Zarafonetis, Muriel C. Meyers, and John A. Penner, who reviewed the manuscript and provided valuable

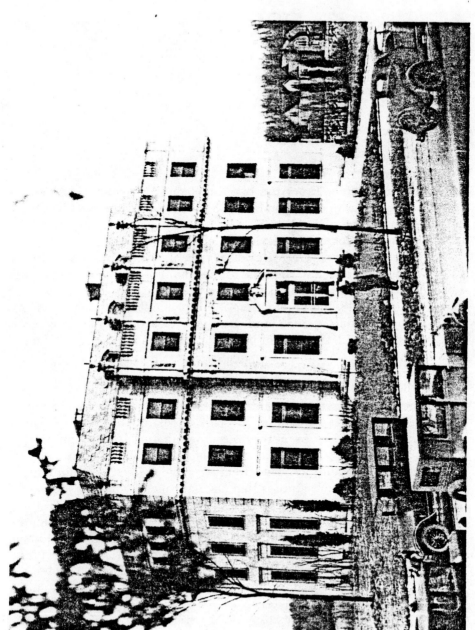

See legend on the opposite page.

suggestions, and the librarians and staff of the Medical Center Library, The University of Michigan. Jean L. Barnard of this library and Janet F. Regier, archives librarian of the Francis A. Countway Library of Medicine in Boston, were especially helpful in locating some of the early historical material on pernicious anemia. Electron microscopic studies of Cabot rings and pernicious anemia marrow cells were performed in collaboration with Dr. Robert H. Gray, School of Public Health, The University of Michigan. Ultrastructural studies of nucleoproteins and nucleic acids isolated from pernicious anemia erythroid precursors were performed in collaboration with Lawrence F. Allard, Department of Materials and Metals Engineering, The University of Michigan, and Mark A. Boroush. I also wish to acknowledge the expert technical assistance of Scott A. Stein, Edgar L. Sherman, Wendell A. Rideout, and James A. Oddo and to thank Jean E. Whipple for typing the manuscript.

This work was supported in part by the Elizabeth Roodvoets Memorial Grant for Cancer Research of the American Cancer Society (CI-79) and by a grant from the National Cancer Institute (USPH CA 14428-01).

Lawrence Kass

The Thomas Henry Simpson Memorial Institute for Medical Research as it appeared at the time of its dedication on February 10, 1927. The building was designed by the noted American architect Albert Kahn. The dedication address was given by Henry A. Christian, M.D., who was the physician-in-chief of the Peter Bent Brigham Hospital at the time.

CONTENTS

CHAPTER 1

HISTORICAL ASPECTS OF PERNICIOUS ANEMIA

Pernicious anemia is a disorder in which atrophic gastritis and resulting achylia gastrica ultimately lead to a deficiency of intrinsic factor. The lack of intrinsic factor leads to malabsorption and subsequently deficiency of vitamin B_{12}. As a result of the deficiency of this vitamin, a characteristic type of macrocytic anemia associated with megaloblastic bone marrow and neuropathy develop. Although the disorder may exhibit spontaneous remissions and exacerbations and is readily curable with vitamin B_{12}, it is fatal if untreated.

Credit for the initial description of what appears to have been pernicious anemia is generally ascribed to J. S. Combe (Fig. 1), a Scottish physician, who described a "history of a case of anaemia" in 1822.[96] Combe concluded that his 47-year-old male patient with a "deadly pale colour" suffered from:

> . . . a species of dyspepsia, and perhaps with propriety; for it is probably owing to some disorder of the digestive and assimilative organs, that its characteristic symptom has its origin, and to the correction of this derangement, we must look for a removal of the disease.

On the basis of this remark, Combe has been credited with the first printed statement that a disorder of the gastrointestinal tract might have had an important etiological relationship to the particular anemia he was describing.

Hall in 1837[185] described certain fatal cases of chlorosis, some of which may have represented pernicious anemia. Likewise, Channing in 1842[90] reported cases of "anhaemia, principally in its connection with the puerperal state and the functional disease of the uterus with cases." Some of these may also have been early accounts of pernicious anemia. Coupland[105] states that Andral in 1823, Piorry in 1841, and

1

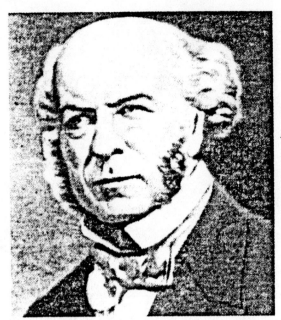

Figure 1. J. S. Combe (1796-1883). (From Medische, W.P. Encyclopaedie 2:219, 1954. Reproduced with permission of Elsevier Publishing Projects, Amsterdam, The Netherlands.)

Figure 2. Thomas Addison (1793-1860). (From Guy's Hospital Gazette 22:520, 1908. Reproduced with permission of Guy's Hospital Gazette, London.)

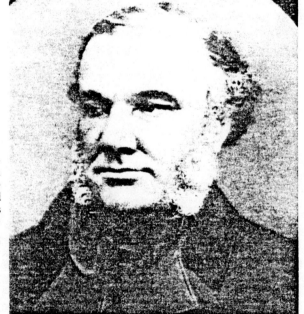

Pearce in 1845 also gave early accounts of severe anemia that may have represented pernicious anemia.

In 1849, Thomas Addison (Fig. 2) described a "remarkable form of anemia" in the *London Medical Gazette*[8] and again recounted his observations of this unusual type of anemia in his treatise on the disease of the "suprarenal capsules"[9] published in 1855. Although Addison believed that this "idiopathic anemia" was related to a disorder of the adrenal glands,[9] and did not mention gastric abnormalities in his account, his report has been regarded as a classic portrayal of an individual with severe pernicious anemia.[104,337]

Barclay[26] described two fatal cases of anemia in 1851 and observed glossitis in one of his patients. Möller[301] in 1851 was also among the first to mention painful glossitis as an important physical finding in certain patients with anemia. In some cases these patients had an infestation with *Diphyllobothrium latum* and may have had findings consistent with vitamin B_{12} deficiency.

In 1860, Austin Flint (Fig. 3) writing on anemia in the *American Medical Times*,[149] described the characteristic physical findings in patients with severe anemia. In what seems to have been a remarkable moment of insight, Flint forecasted an etiological relationship between this severe anemia and gastric atrophy:

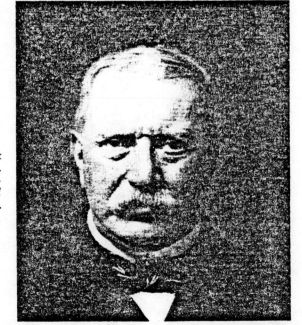

Figure 3. Austin Flint (1812-1886). (From Flint, A. *Collected Essays and Articles on Physiology and Medicine (1855-1902)*, vol. 1. Appleton - Century - Crofts, New York, 1903.)

I suspect that in these cases there exists degenerative disease of the glandular tubuli of the stomach. . . . Nor is it difficult to see how fatal anaemia must follow an amount of degenerative disease reducing the amount of gastric juice so far that the assimilation of food is rendered wholly inadequate to the wants of the body. I shall be ready to claim the merit of this idea when the difficult and laborious researches of some one have shown it to be correct.

During the period between 1850 and 1880, technical advances in the enumeration of formed elements of the blood and morphological observations regarding the origin of erythrocytes were made. Although these discoveries may not have appeared to have had a direct relationship to pernicious anemia at the time, when viewed in their historical context they seem to be a part of a growing framework of knowledge regarding the production of erythrocytes and the detection and evaluation of anemia.

Karl Vierordt (Fig. 4) in 1852[409] was the first to perform actual counts of erythrocytes, using instruments that by today's standards would be considered rudimentary. Hayem and Nachet[193] in 1875 improved Vierordt's somewhat lengthy and impractical method by devising a new type of capillary pipette and counting chamber and using squares ruled on the eyepiece of the microscope to encompass the erythrocytes in the field and provide a basis for enumeration. In 1877, Gowers[173] modified Hayem and Nachet's method by engraving the counting squares on the counting chamber (hemacytometer) itself, thereby permitting erythrocyte counts to be performed with any microscope. Since, at the time, assessment of anemia was made primarily

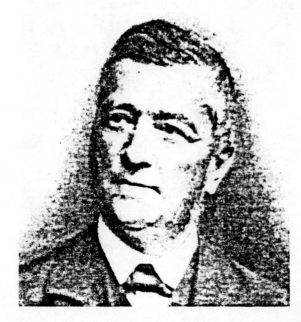

Figure 4. Karl Vierordt (1818-1884). (From Pagel, J. *Biographisches Lexicon hervorragender Aerzte des neunzehnten Jahrhunderts.* Urban & Schwarzenberg, Berlin, 1901, p. 1767.)

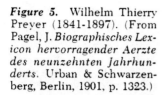

Figure 5. Wilhelm Thierry Preyer (1841-1897). (From Pagel, J. *Biographisches Lexicon hervorragender Aerzte des neunzehnten Jahrhunderts.* Urban & Schwarzenberg, Berlin, 1901, p. 1323.)

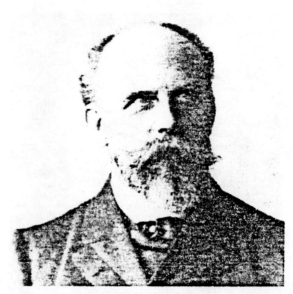

by inspection of peripheral blood films and smears, these technical advancements permitting actual quantitation of erythrocytes facilitated a more objective measurement of the degree of anemia than previously possible.

Further technical advances in hematology at the time that ultimately contributed to the increasing body of information about pernicious anemia were the development of various techniques to measure hemoglobin. Funke[158] discovered hemoglobin in 1851, and Wilhelm Preyer (Fig. 5) in 1871[333] wrote the first monograph on hemoglobin and described various spectroscopic, colorimetric, and chemical methods for determining this substance.

Also interspersed among the clinical accounts of pernicious anemia was the important observation of Ernst Neumann (Fig. 6), who in 1868 was the first to report that erythrocytes in the peripheral blood originated from nucleated erythroid precursors in the bone marrow.[310] The significance of Neumann's conclusion that erythrogenesis occurred in the marrow was appreciated by Cohnheim, Osler, and Ehrlich, and these authors referred to Neumann's observations in their own reports regarding the marrow origin of pernicious anemia erythroid precursors approximately ten years later.

The next phases in the history of pernicious anemia were the contributions of the Swiss physician, Anton Biermer (Fig. 7). In 1868, Biermer[44] presented a preliminary report regarding the effects of severe anemia on the heart and vessels. He mentioned cases of idio-

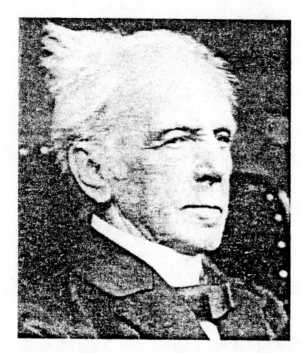

Figure 6. Ernst Neumann (1834-1918). (From the pictorial archives of the New York Academy of Medicine Library. To the best of the author's knowledge, this is the only published portrait of Neumann.)

Figure 7. Anton Biermer (1827-1892). (From Schweiz. Med. Wschr. *64*(23) (front), 1934. Reproduced with permission of Schwabe & Co., Basel, Switzerland.)

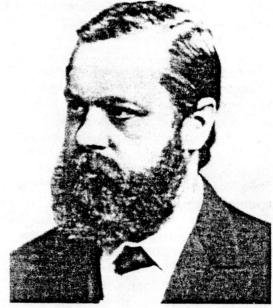

pathic and secondary anemia in middle-age patients who became anemic because of blood loss and chronic diarrhea, but he did not use the term *progressive pernicious anemia* in this initial and fragmentary account.

In 1872, Biermer[45] gave the name *progressive pernicious anemia* to a "peculiar form" of anemia. Reference is made to the earlier report of 1868 as being a preliminary report of this progressive pernicious anemia.[45,169] Although the name *progressive pernicious anemia* was a particularly colorful term, it is uncertain whether Biermer actually described true pernicious anemia at all. Modern translations of Biermer's account suggest that his cases were probably heterogeneous and that some represented the anemia of pregnancy (perhaps secondary to folate deficiency), the anemia of chronic renal failure, and perhaps the anemia of chronic disease. Biermer's oldest patient, a 52-year-old man, may have actually had true pernicious anemia, but it is uncertain.

Descriptions of gastric disorders began to appear in the literature almost simultaneously with the initial clinical descriptions of pernicious anemia. Samuel Fenwick (Fig. 8) in 1870[144] was the first to describe gastric atrophy. He observed that in a specimen of the stomach obtained at necropsy from one of his patients who had pallor, dyspepsia, and "anemia," the gastric juice did not possess its usual proteolytic activity. It is possible that Fenwick's patient may have also had pernicious anemia since he is described as being "pale" and having "anemia," in addition to having atrophic gastritis. A reproduc-

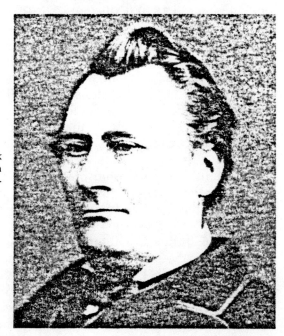

Figure 8. Samuel Fenwick (1821-1902). (Reproduced with permission of The National Portrait Gallery, London.)

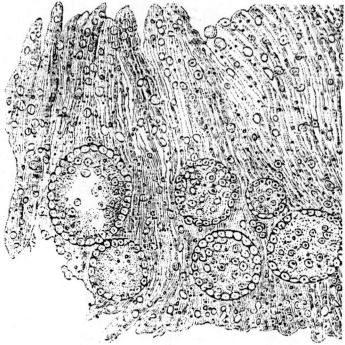

Figure 9. Line drawing illustrating atrophy of gastric tubules from Fenwick's 1870 paper.

tion of a line drawing showing gastric tubular atrophy from Fenwick's original paper of 1870 is illustrated in Figure 9.

A wave of enthusiasm swept both American and continental physicians following Biermer's initial description of pernicious anemia. William Pepper (Fig. 10) in 1875 described "progressive pernicious anemia or anaematosis" in which he reported three cases of what appear to have been pernicious anemia.[324] In the third case of a 50-year-old man, Pepper gave the first account of the appearance of the bone marrow in pernicious anemia. Although Pepper wrote that "there existed extreme hyperplasia of the marrow with production of lymphoid cells," it is conceivable that these "lymphoid cells" may have actually been erythroid precursors. Howard[217] in 1876 also described several cases of progressive pernicious anemia and gave early accounts of the gross and microscopic descriptions of the bone marrow.

In 1876, Julius Cohnheim (Fig. 11) wrote a still more detailed description of the marrow in pernicious anemia.[95] Cohnheim was the first to recognize that the hyperplasia of cells in the bone marrow of patients with pernicious anemia was due to markedly increased numbers of erythroid precursors. Cohnheim also referred to Neumann's[310] discovery that erythrogenesis occurred in the bone marrow and stated

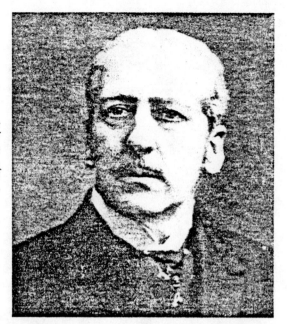

Figure 10. William Pepper (1843-1898). (From *Builders of American Medicine*. George Wahr, Ann Arbor, 1932, p. 135. Reproduced with permission of George Wahr Publishing Co., Ann Arbor, Michigan.)

that a similar phenomenon occurred in pernicious anemia. William Osler (Fig. 12) included pernicious anemia among his widespread medical interests and prolific literary output. Osler and Gardner[315] and Osler[316] in 1877 wrote early descriptions of the appearance of the bone marrow in pernicious anemia, and they, as well as Cohnheim, were

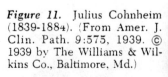

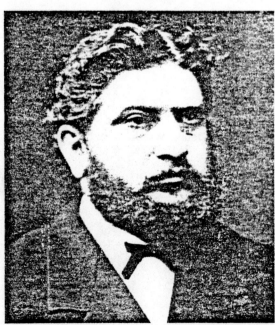

Figure 11. Julius Cohnheim (1839-1884). (From Amer. J. Clin. Path. 9:575, 1939. © 1939 by The Williams & Wilkins Co., Baltimore, Md.)

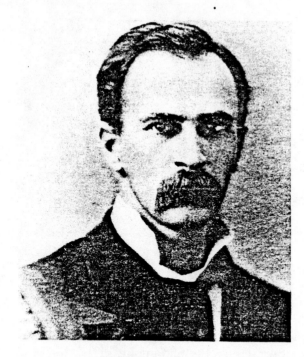

Figure 12. William Osler (1848-1919) as a young professor at McGill University. (From Cushing, H. *The Life of Sir William Osler,* vol. 1 (frontispiece), Oxford University Press, Oxford, 1925. Reproduced with permission of Oxford University Press, Oxford, England.)

Figure 13. Hermann Eichhorst (1849-1929). (From Deutsch. Med. Wschr. *30*:608, 1904. Reproduced with permission of Georg Thieme Verlag, Stuttgart, Germany.)

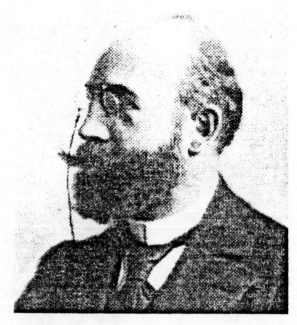

among the first to note the extreme erythroid hyperplasia of the bone marrow.

Descriptions of the bone marrow in pernicious anemia seem to have ushered in the next phase in the history of this disorder. During this period peripheral blood erythrocyte abnormalities and the megaloblast were described. Hermann Eichhorst (Fig. 13) in 1876 was the first to describe the microcyte in pernicious anemia,[134] and he believed that the microcyte was a characteristic and diagnostic finding in this disorder. Microcytes as illustrated in Eichhorst's 1878 monograph on anemia[135] are reproduced in Figure 14. Heinrich Quincke (Fig. 15)

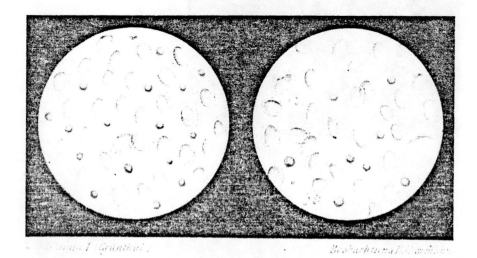

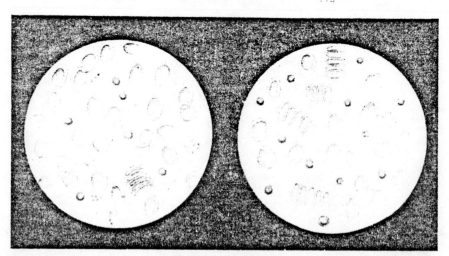

Figure 14. Reproduction of plate from Eichhorst's 1878 monograph on pernicious anemia, illustrating microcytes in the peripheral blood of patients with pernicious anemia.

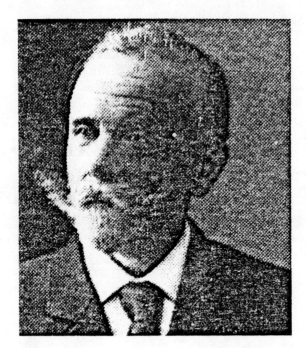

Figure 15. Heinrich Quincke (1842-1922). (From
Deutsch. Med. Wschr.
30:608, 1904. Reproduced
with permission of Georg
Thieme Verlag, Stuttgart,
Germany.)

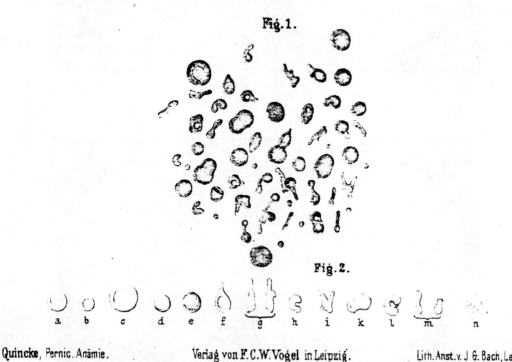

Fig.1.

Fig.2.

Quincke, Pernic. Anämie.   Verlag von F.C.W.Vogel in Leipzig.   Lith.Anst.v.J G.Bach,Leipzig

Figure 16. Reproduction of plate from Quincke's 1877 publication illustrating misshapen erythrocytes (poikilocytes) from the peripheral blood of a patient with pernicious anemia. (From Deutsch. Arch. Klin. Med. 20:1, 1877.)

also contributed to the early knowledge of the morphological abnormalities of erythrocytes in pernicious anemia. In 1876-1877, Quincke[338-340] was the first to describe the extreme variation in shape of the erythrocytes in the peripheral blood of patients with pernicious anemia. Quincke called this variation "poikilocytosis."[340] A reproduction of these poikilocytes from Quincke's 1877 paper[340] is shown in Figure 16. George Hayem (Fig. 17) who had devised a method for counting red blood cells in 1875[193] wrote extensively about the morphological abnormalities of erythrocytes in various types of anemias. Although Laache[257] is generally credited with the first description of the macrocyte in pernicious anemia, it was actually Hayem in 1877 who first described *globules géants* or giant erythrocytes in the blood of patients with severe pernicious anemia.[194,195]

In a detailed and lucid account written in 1879, Paul Ehrlich[128] described a triacid stain that could be used to differentiate various types of cells in the blood. As hematology in general advanced as a result of Ehrlich's discovery of these staining reactions, knowledge of the morphological characteristics of cells in pernicious anemia also became clarified. In 1880, Ehrlich (Fig. 18) applied his cytoplasmic and nuclear stain to the large nucleated erythroid precursors in the blood of pernicious anemia patients.[129,130] Ehrlich called these cells "megaloblasts."[129] He credited Hayem[194,195] with the first recognition of the "giant blood corpuscles," presumably large macroovalocytes and giant macrocytes, in the blood of patients with pernicious anemia and stated that megaloblasts were the precursors of these giant erythrocytes. In 1883, Sören Laache (Fig. 19) in another of the early mono-

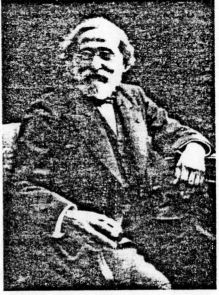

Figure 17. Georges Hayem (1841-1933). (From Bull. Acad. Méd. *110*:149, 1933. Reproduced with permission of Masson et Cie, Paris.)

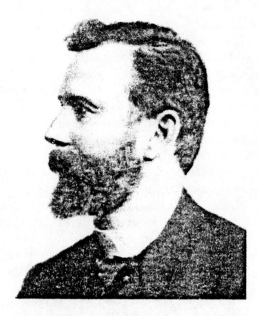

Figure 18. Paul Ehrlich (1854-1915), aged about 40. (From München. Med. Wschr. *61*:575, 1914. Reproduced with permission of J. F. Lehmanns Verlag, Munich.)

graphs on pernicious anemia,[257] was the first to illustrate macrocytes in this disorder, although Hayem[194,195] had probably described these cells earlier in 1877. Reproductions of macrocytes from Laache's original 1883 monograph[257] are shown in Figure 20.

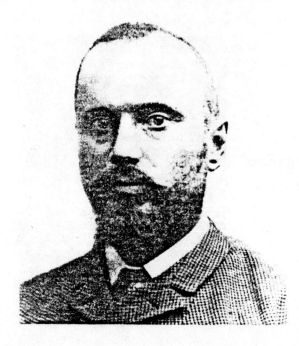

Figure 19. Sören Laache (1854-1941). (From Acta Med. Scand. *108*:151, 1941. Reproduced with permission of Acta Medica Scandinavica.)

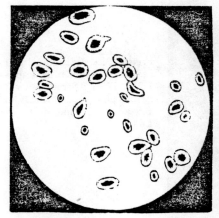
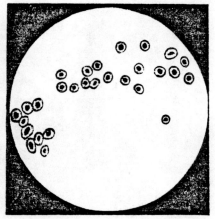
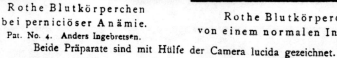

Rothe Blutkörperchen
bei perniciöser Anämie.
Pat. No. 4. Anders Ingebretsen.

Rothe Blutkörperchen
von einem normalen Individuum.

Beide Präparate sind mit Hülfe der Camera lucida gezeichnet.

Figure 20. Reproduction of plate from Laache's original 1883 monograph on pernicious anemia, illustrating macrocytes (left) in the peripheral blood.

Cahn and von Mering[67] in 1886 were among the first to systematically study the physiology of the stomach in various disorders and actually determine the acid content of gastric secretions. They concluded that "in case of fever or severe anemia, hydrochloric acid may occasionally be missing." These authors also proposed an etiological relationship between achlorhydria and anemia.

MacKenzie[282] in 1878 and Addison's pupil Pye-Smith[337] in 1882 gave early accounts of pernicious anemia. MacKenzie[282] was one of the

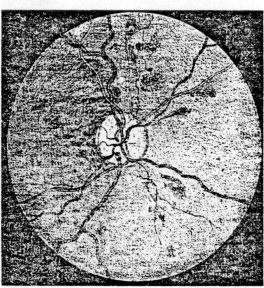

Figure 21. Retinal hemorrhages in pernicious anemia, as illustrated by MacKenzie in 1878.

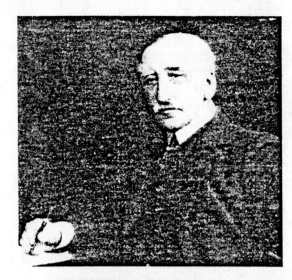

Figure 22. William Hunter (1861-1937). (From Lancet *1*:235, 1937. Reproduced with permission of The Lancet and Bassano and Vandyk Studios, London.)

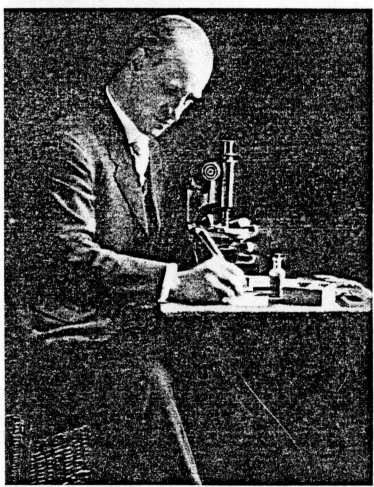

Figure 23. Richard C. Cabot (1868-1939) at his microscope in an early photograph. (Reproduced with permission of the Francis A. Countway Library of Medicine, Harvard University, Boston.)

16

first to illustrate retinal hemorrhages in patients with pernicious anemia, as reproduced in Figure 21. William Hunter[218,219] and others [4,105,265,356] also wrote extensively on pernicious anemia at the time. Based in part on pathological findings of extensive hepatic hemosiderosis, Hunter (Fig. 22) championed the viewpoint that pernicious anemia was primarily a hemolytic disorder.

In 1898, Richard C. Cabot (Fig. 23), a prominent Boston physician, wrote a textbook of hematology[64] in which he described the clinical and morphological features of pernicious anemia in detail. Cabot also described and illustrated the staining properties of the nucleus of the megaloblast in his book (Chapter 10), and in 1900[65] he reported the clinical and blood findings in 110 cases of pernicious anemia. In 1903, Cabot[66] reported an unusual type of ring-shaped inclusion in erythrocytes obtained from the peripheral blood of patients with pernicious anemia, lead poisoning, and leukemia. Cabot was uncertain of the derivation of these "ring bodies," now referred to as Cabot rings, but speculated that they might be nuclear remnants. A figure from Cabot's original 1903 paper describing and illustrating these ring bodies is reproduced in Figure 24.

As more precise techniques for quantitation entered the field of hematology, certain of the earlier morphological observations of erythrocyte abnormalities in pernicious anemia could be studied more critically. Capps[72] in 1903 was one of the first to perform actual volumetric measurements of erythrocytes in pernicious anemia and confirmed Hayem's and Laache's original morphological observations that these erythrocytes were larger than normal. Shortly thereafter in 1905, and perhaps as a result of improvements in staining techniques, Ehrlich and Lazarus[133] described the morphological characteristics of the megaloblast in detail. They noted that the nucleus of the megaloblast

. . . is especially differentiated from the nucleus of the normoblasts by a much less marked affinity for the nuclear stains—in fact, this affinity is sometimes so slight that the inexpert may fail to notice the nucleus.

This remarkable morphological observation at the time seems to have presaged present-day theories of the pathogenesis of the megaloblastic lesion (Chapter 10) based on abnormalities in the biosynthesis of both DNA[30-34,292,342,398] and histones.[238-240,242]

For many years, the intense interest in the erythroid abnormalities of pernicious anemia dominated scientific investigations of this disorder. Although variations in leukocyte counts had been mentioned by several authors as occurring in pernicious anemia[64,133], qualitative abnormalities of leukocytes did not receive much attention until 1907 when the German hematologist Joseph Arneth (Fig. 25), in a monograph on disorders of the blood,[18] first described the now-familiar abnormalities of the polymorphonuclear leukocyte in perni-

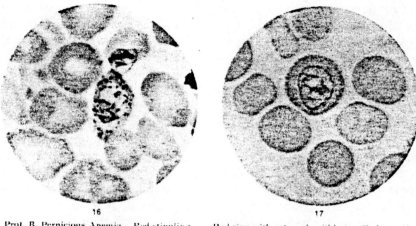

16
Prof. B. Pernicious Anemia. Red stippling
and rings, partially extra cellular.

Red ring with net work within it. Red stippling,
Mrs. B. Pernicious Anemia.

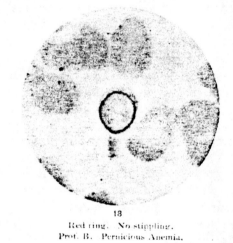

18
Red ring. No stippling.
Prof. B. Pernicious Anemia.

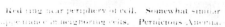

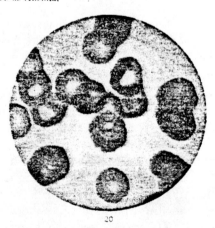

19
Red ring near periphery of cell. Somewhat similar
appearance in neighboring cells. Pernicious Anemia.

20
Lead Poisoning. No rings. Red ring
Apparently but not really extra cellular.

Figure 24. Reproduction of plate from Cabot's 1903 article describing ring bodies in
pernicious anemia erythrocytes. (J. Med. Res. 9:15, 1903.)

cious anemia. Arneth reported and illustrated both the increased size of the polymorphonuclear leukocyte and the increased numbers of nuclear lobulations in this cell in two patients with severe pernicious anemia. One of the two original line drawings from Arneth's 1907 monograph[18] showing the "shift to the right" with the large, hyper-

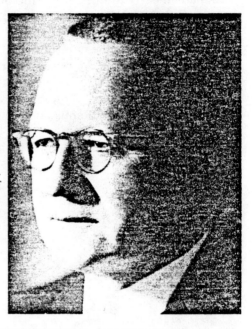

Figure 25. Joseph Arneth (1873-1955). (From Arneth, J. *Gesammelte Qualitativ-haematologische Untersuchungen 1936-1944.* J. A. Barth Verlag, Frankfurt, 1944. Reproduced with permission of J. A. Barth.) The diagram is a reproduction of Arneth's original illustration of abnormalities in size and nuclear hypersegmentation ("shift to the right") of polymorphonuclear leukocytes from the peripheral blood of a patient with severe pernicious anemia. (From Arneth, J. *Diagnose und Therapie der Anämien.* Stuber, Würzburg, Germany, 1907.)

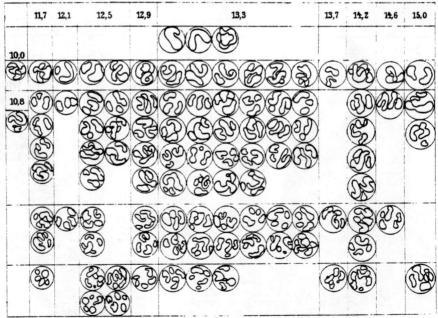

Anmerk.: Dieses Blutbild ist das am stärksten „nach Rechts" entwickelte, das bis jetzt überhaupt von dem Verfasser angetroffen wurde.

segmented polymorphonuclear leukocytes in pernicious anemia is reproduced in Figure 25. Arneth's original observations were later popularized by Cooke,[97] who called the large hypersegmented neutrophils "macropolycytes."

Although he was a renowned cardiologist, Samuel A. Levine (Fig. 26) had an early interest in pernicious anemia, as did other physicians at the Peter Bent Brigham Hospital in Boston in the early part of the twentieth century.[384,387] Levine and Ladd[273] in 1921 published one of the earliest and most complete studies documenting a firm relationship between achlorhydria and pernicious anemia. They also noted that achlorhydria could be present for years before the blood abnormalities appeared and "possibly always antedates them." Levine and Ladd found that pernicious anemia exhibited a familial tendency, an

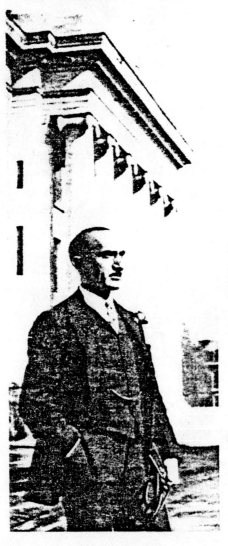

Figure 26. Samuel A. Levine (1891-1966) in 1925. (From Medical World News 6(10):55, 1965. Reproduced with permission of the Peter Bent Brigham Hospital, Boston.)

increased frequency in "English-speaking people" and Scandinavians, and often had peripheral blood eosinophilia as a prominent feature. Hurst[221] in 1923 also stressed the importance of the etiological relationship of achlorhydria to the development of pernicious anemia. Bloomfield and Keefer[50] in 1927 performed extensive studies of gastric function in various disorders including pernicious anemia and confirmed the earlier observations of achlorhydria in this disorder.

Actual scientific experimentation regarding factors responsible for the pathogenesis of severe anemia began with the work of Hooper and Whipple[215] in 1918. These investigators showed that blood regeneration in dogs made anemic by bleeding was particularly rapid on a meat diet, and they were among the first to implicate dietary factors in the formation of blood. Whipple et al.[424] in 1920 found that cooked liver, lean beef, or heart led to rapid blood regeneration in anemic dogs and stressed the value of liver in particular as a potent hematopoietic substance.

In 1922, Whipple[425] stated that increased stercobilin production in pernicious anemia resulted from increased production of this substance rather than from increased destruction of erythrocytes. Whipple proposed that a factor, presumably dietary and responsible for the

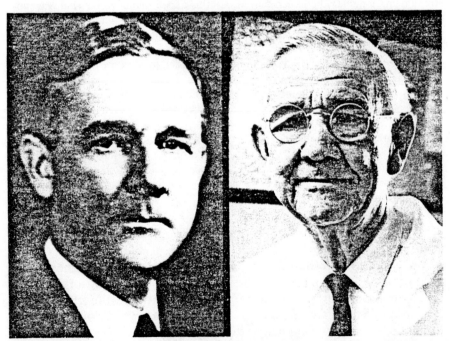

Figure 27. *Left:* George H. Whipple (1878–1976) in 1934. (Reproduced with permission of the Nobel Foundation, Stockholm, Sweden.) *Right:* George H. Whipple in a photograph taken in 1972 at age 94. (Courtesy of the University of Rochester School of Medicine and Dentistry, Rochester, New York. Photograph by Louis Ouzer.)

production of material from which the "stroma" of erythrocytes were formed in the bone marrow in pernicious anemia, might be lacking in this disorder. In additional experiments in 1925, Whipple and Robscheit-Robbins[426,427] and Robscheit-Robbins and Whipple[349] found that ". . . liver feeding in these severe anemias remains the most potent factor for the sustained production of hemoglobin and erythrocytes."[349] They also noted that " . . . even in complex anemias (human pernicious anemia, anemia with nephritis and cancer cachexia) food factors deserve serious considerations in the clinical management of the blood condition."[427]

In a recent interview,[306] George H. Whipple (Fig. 27) recalled some of his early efforts to delineate the role of nutritional substances in the treatment of anemia:

> Out in California, I was given quarters in an old veterinary building where I conducted research on the influence of diet in bile pigment output. When I realized that hemoglobin was a factor, I began intensive study of hemoglobin production and, after testing various food material, found that liver was the most important agent.
>
> At that time a Dr. Charles Hooper was working with me, and he wanted to test a liver extract on pernicious anemia patients. Dr. Hooper's extract was an alcoholic, fat-free preparation that he gave subcutaneously to three patients; all showed remissions and greatly elevated hemoglobin levels.
>
> However, the other clinicians laughed him out of the wards, telling him that the remissions were spontaneous and of no significance. Hooper was a shy, sensitive young man, and this ridicule led him to quit this experimental work. That was most unfortunate, because the extract almost certainly contained the potent B_{12} factor from the liver, and the cure for pernicious anemia might have been discovered in 1918. . . .
>
> In the spring of 1921, I was once more persuaded to pack my bags, this time for Rochester, N.Y., to found a new medical school at the university there. I brought my 40 dogs with me and continued my research while acting as dean of the school and hiring a staff. Much of the laboratory work was done by Dr. Frieda Robbins, who moved from California with us.
>
> By that time, I had published several papers showing the beneficial effect of liver on dogs in whom we induced anemia by bleeding. At Rochester I continued with investigations of liver fractions and muscle hemoglobin and standardized a liver fraction that was potent in secondary anemia. Eli Lilly marketed the fraction and supported our work. . . .

Running concurrently with the developments in and discoveries of the gastric, hematological, and neurological manifestations of pernicious anemia and the role of nutritional factors in the pathogenesis of anemia was the increasing recognition of the young erythrocyte forms, or reticulocytes, in the peripheral blood and the growing appreciation of their significance as indicators of erythropoietic activity in the bone marrow. The use of the reticulocyte rise as an indicator of response to hematopoietic substances seemed to attain almost instantaneous importance in Minot and Murphy's report in 1926.[298] Yet, cells that were probably reticulocytes had been described by Ehrlich many years earlier,[131,132] although he believed that these cells were degenerating erythrocytes.

The suggestion that these erythrocytes might be young red cells rather than degenerating red cells was made by Theobald Smith[378] in 1891 in his account of changes in erythrocytes in the "pernicious anemia" of Texas cattle fever, a tickborne disease caused by the protozoan *Boophilus annulatus*. Smith found "unfinished or embryonic corpuscles" in the blood of these animals. The tinctorial properties of these "embryonic corpuscles" seem identical to those described earlier in "degenerating" erythrocytes by Ehrlich.[131,132] In 1913, Pepper and Peet[323] reflected the growing awareness of the significance of the reticulocyte by observing that an "increase in the number of reticulated cells is evidence of unusual activity in blood production."

George R. Minot (Fig. 28) was probably aware of the role of the reticulocyte at least ten years prior to the dramatic announcement of the efficacy of liver therapy for pernicious anemia in 1926. In 1916, Lee, Minot, and Vincent,[267] in their study of splenectomy in pernicious anemia, stated that:

> The percentage of reticulated red cells may perhaps be taken as a measure of the hemopoietic activity of the bone marrow. . . . A high percentage of reticulated cells probably indicates an increased activity of the part of the bone marrow that produces red cells.

These authors observed that increased reticulocyte counts were the

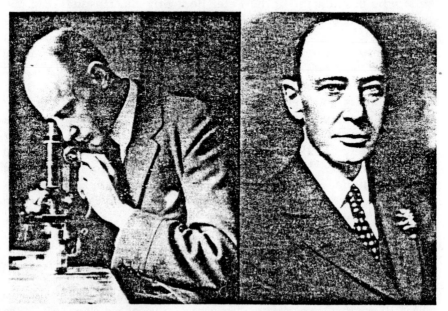

Figure 28. Left: George R. Minot at his microscope in a 1917 photograph. *Right:* George R. Minot (1885-1950) in 1934. (Reproduced with permission of the Nobel Foundation, Stockholm, Sweden.)

forerunners of increased red blood cell counts, and they stressed that continuous and meticulous observations of reticulocytes over a period of time were needed to assess bone marrow erythropoietic activity accurately. Thus, with the growing awareness of the significance of the reticulocyte and the implications of a rising reticulocyte count, the stage had been set for Minot and Murphy to utilize the reticulocyte response in their investigations of the effect of liver in pernicious anemia.

Liver entered the pernicious anemia story at this point as a result of several factors. Minot and Murphy were both aware of Whipple's studies showing the hematopoietic effects of liver in anemic dogs. Based on Whipple's observations, they recommended to certain of their office patients who had anemia that they include liver in their diets. According to Minot, liver was fed to several such patients with pernicious anemia in 1924 and 1925, but the results were inconclusive,[300] perhaps in part because these patients had been followed in an outpatient office setting and their responses to liver were not carefully documented in a controlled environment. In several patients with pernicious anemia, however, Minot and Murphy observed that the inclusion of liver in the diet did seem to have a beneficial effect. In one particular instance, a patient with pernicious anemia who ate unusually large amounts of liver seemed to do unusually well.[306]

Based upon these sporadic but seemingly beneficial responses, it was proposed that the effects of liver therapy in pernicious anemia be investigated systematically in a series of patients.[306] These patients were to be hospitalized at the Peter Bent Brigham Hospital (Fig. 29) so that their hematological and clinical responses to liver could be meticulously observed with daily physical examinations and serial blood counts. The reticulocyte count as an indicator of erythropoietic activity of the bone marrow, as recognized earlier by Minot and others, was an integral part of the hematological assessment.

In January and February of 1926, the beneficial effects of liver were convincingly documented for the first time in a 44-year-old Nova Scotian machinist with severe untreated pernicious anemia. In a recent interview[306] in 1972 and in his monograph on pernicious anemia published in 1939,[305] William P. Murphy (Fig. 30) recounted some of his early experiences and observations on this first patient with pernicious anemia treated in the hospital with liver and documented to have a hematological response:

> . . . This patient, a man in his late forties, was critically ill and partially comatose, with a red blood cell count of around 800,000. In spite of the fact that he was in a partial coma, I was able to explain to him what we were doing and that liver might be distinctly useful to him.
>
> We had found that improvement could be demonstrated in pernicious anemia patients by counting the number of reticulocytes, or young red blood cells, in the stained smear. We also found that if a patient were fed half a pound of liver per day, it would take about five days to register an increase in the reticulocyte count.

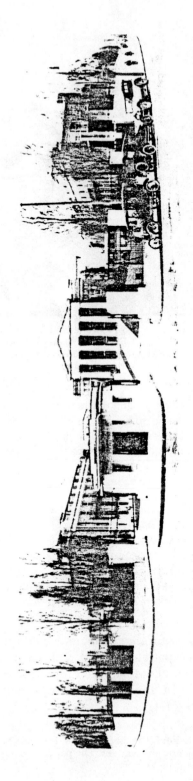

Figure 29. The Peter Bent Brigham Hospital, Boston, in a panoramic view taken from Brigham Circle on May 20, 1920. A model of innovative hospital design at the time, it was opened in 1913. The white-columned administration building is seen in the center. At the far left are the patient pavilions, connected to the main hospital by a long hallway or "pike" which is not visible in the picture. (Photograph reproduced with permission of the Peter Bent Brigham Hospital, Boston.)

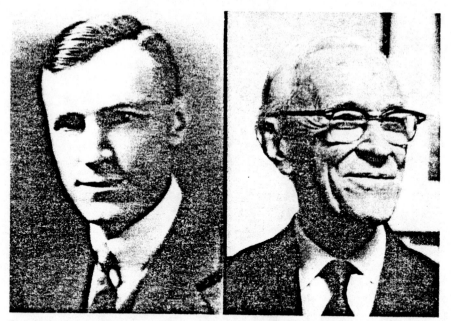

Figure 30. Left: William P. Murphy (1892-   ) in 1934. (Reproduced with permission of the Nobel Foundation, Stockholm, Sweden.) *Right:* William P. Murphy in 1972. (Reproduced with permission of Joe Baker-Medical World News, New York.)

But this man seemed to be more ill on the fifth day of treatment. . . . I stayed up very late that night, trying to decide whether to give him a transfusion or to give him the liver—it was a miserable night. However, around midnight I noticed that his reticulocyte count had increased slightly, and that gave me the courage to withhold transfusion and go on with the liver. . . .

Although this patient had previously been eating other things such as vegetables along with the liver, during those five days it was strictly liver. When I saw his reticulocyte count go up, I went home and collapsed into bed, slept very poorly, and was back at the hospital by seven o'clock the next morning.

I approached his room with fear and trembling, and cautiously peeked around the corner to see if he was still alive. To my great surprise and relief he sat up in bed and cheerfully asked, "What time is breakfast?"

I then discovered that his reticulocyte count had reached its maximum, and I felt confident that he would survive in excellent condition. He not only survived but lived for many years.[306]

By courtesy of the Peter Bent Brigham Hospital, excerpts from the actual hospital chart of this first patient treated with liver in January and February of 1926 and documented to have a hematological response are herein reproduced.* In this hospital chart, the liver diet is referred to as the "high purine diet."

---

*I am deeply indebted to the Peter Bent Brigham Hospital, Boston, Massachusetts, for permitting me to reproduce this historical document. The patient's name and hospital number have been obliterated to ensure anonymity.

PETER BENT BRIGHAM HOSPITAL
MEDICAL SERVICE

Date Jan 14, 1926   Hosp. No.

Name   Med. No.

Residence   O. D. D. No.
                  Boston, Mass.
Birthplace   Canada   Age 14   M__M. S. D.   White or Colored

Occupation   Machinist

Date of Adm.   Jan 14, 1926   Patient's Physician, Dr. E.J.Wagner,

Date of Disch.   Feb. 21,1926   Address   240 Highland Ave., Somerville, Mass.
                  Improved   Dr. A.N.Curtiss, P.B.B.H. O.D.D.

Address—Parents or Friends
                  Aunt__

                  Pr__

Transfer to or from surgical   Surgical Number

Re-Entry   See   *Medical #*

Diagnosis PERNICIOUS ANEMIA (13-68.1)   (C.F.)

Complications
Complaint   "Weakness and Shortness of breath".

F. H.   Father died of "cancer of the esophagus" at the age of 80 Mother aged
                  55 is living and well. One sister living. Her condition is unknown to the
          patient.   The patient tells of no family history of diabetes, gout, tuberculosis,
          hemophilia, arthritis, or diseases of the circulatory, respiratory, digestive,
          renal, nervous or muscular systems

Marital   Not married

Social History   The patient is a single machinist who occupies one room in a boarding
          house. He does not pay rent while in the hospital. He has an aged mother who
          is apparently only partly dependent upon him. During his disease other folks will
          take care of her.   The patient has no home or place suited for convalescence. He
          is of German descent, was born in Nova Scotia. He came to this country at the
          age of 14 and has no language difficulties. He is fairly well educated and is
          intelligent enough to follow diet instructions and can pay for the same. On
          a restricted diet he will be able to carry on his regular work. No emotional
          factors in the patient's home at the present time.

Habits   The patient usually works eight or nine hours a day. Sleeps seven or
          eight. He was interested in labor problems, cooperative movement and to a slight
          degree, in politics. He has never used any drugs, alcohol, tea or patent medicines
          Coffee—3 cups every day. No tobacco or alcohol

Occupation   Machinist at the Electric Heating Co. Boston. The patient has been

Chart continued on the following page

-2-

PETER BENT BRIGHAM HOSPITAL
MEDICAL SERVICE

NAME _____   WARD ____   F_2 MED. NO.

working along this line for 25 years. His work in this kind of industry is
irregular, three or four months of work are followed by an interval of idleness
for one or two months or more. He has never worked nights. His work has never
been very tiresome.

P. H.   The patient was born in Nova Scotia and came to the Boston at the age of
12 where he has spent most of his life. He has had chicken pox diphtheria,
measles, and scarlet fever in childhood. Pneumonia at the age of 12. He
had pains in both shoulder, for a number of years, without swelling of these
joints and without noticeable fever. No history of whooping cough, influenza,
tonsillitis, chorea, pleurisy, malaria, or typhoid fever. No association with
tuberculosis or other diseases. At the age of 24 he had some obscure disease
with fever of 102-103°. He was admitted to the B.C.H. at that time, where he was
under observation for 17 days. He was discharged entirely well. In general,
the patient has always been in good health

          Previous Hospital Entries --B.C.H. 22 years ago and the same hospital
in Dec. 1925 to Jan 1926, for weakness.

          Injuries --The patient had his big toe crushed some years ago. His left
eye was also injured by a file. This was followed by a diminution of vision in
that eye

          Operations--None.

          Head--No headaches or trauma. Eyes--Glasses since the injury--see
Injuries No inflammation. The patient's vision has been failing somewhat
during the last year. At the present time he can hardly read a paper. Ears--No
loss of hearing, pain or discharge. Nose--No head colds, discharge, epistaxis
or symptoms of obstruction. Teeth--The upper and lower molars, first and second
are missing. Numerous fillings with silver. Throat--No tonsillitis, sore
throat, hoarseness or sore mouth

          Cardio-respiratory--No pain in the chest, palpitation, dyspnea, cough,
sputum, hemoptysis, or night sweats, except for some slight dyspnea on exertion

          Gastro-intestinal--The patient has his meals at regular intervals.
His appetite is good. He has always had a tendency to be constipated. His
bowels move once every other day and not infrequently, every three days. There
is no nausea, gas, vomiting, hematemesis, distress, colic, icterus, diarrhoea,
bloody, tarry, or clay colored stools. No hemorrhoids.

-3-

PETER BENT BRIGHAM HOSPITAL
MEDICAL SERVICE
NAME   WARD   F-2   MED. NO

Genito-urinary—No dysuria, hematuria, smoky urine, pyuria, retention, incontinence, frequency or nocturia. No history of syphilis or soft chancre. Gonorrhoea without complications and with complete recovery at 25.

Neuro-muscular—The patient is of an even temperament. There is no history of vertigo, fainting, twitching, spasms, anesthesia, paresthesia, ataxia, girdle, shooting, muscular or joint pains. The memory of the patient has always been good. He is worried about his present condition and there is just cause for this worry

Weight— 46 kg. on admission: He thinks he had lost about 15 lbs. during the P.I.

Personality—The patient apparently does not appreciate the seriousness of his condition. He seems to be a conscientious individual and the history as given is reliable

P. I.   The P. I. began approximately in June 1924 with a sensation of distress in the epigastrium. This was soon followed by a disagreeable sensation in the lower part of the abdomen which the patient describes as an intense quiver. This was definitely related to meals always appearing after breakfast, lunch and lasting for a few hours. His appetite which was fairly good up to the onset of the P. I. grew worse every day. About three months later the patient developed a very intense sore tongue which was particularly marked while he was taking food. He also felt that he was getting weaker and around August 1924 he was obliged to stop working. During the time he lost from 10-15 pounds in weight, became very pale and finally was unable to even move without causing complete exhaustion.

In Feb 1925, that is nine months after the onset of the disease, the patient noticed an almost sudden and remarkable improvement in his condition
                                        to his
He "picked up" this normal weight, color and strength. (He attributes this improvement to sauerkraut, of which he consumed a great deal at that time) In May 1925 he felt so strong as to be able to start to work again. He resumed his old occupation in an Electric heating Co. where he remained until June 1925, working eight hours daily. During this period of improvement, the patient did not, however, regain his normal appetite. His tongue was sore but less so than previously.

In June 1925 he again began to have discomfort in the epigastrium.

Chart continued on the following page

L4_

PETER BENT BRIGHAM HOSPITAL
MEDICAL SERVICE

NAME

WARD   F_2 MED. NO

the soreness of the tongue increased in severity and he lost his appetite
and some weight during a period of two or three months, the exact amount not
known. In August 1925 owing to weakness he had to quit his job. He was advised
to go to Canada where he remained from September to Dec. without any improvement
in his condition. For the last few months he has become progressively short of
breath on exertion and has begun to have numbness in his fingers and feet.

The first week in Dec. 1925 he was admitted to the B.C.H. He
remained there three weeks and was discharged unimproved about a week ago
During the last seven days he was so weak that he could hardly cross the room
He now comes in for further treatment

P. E.   The patient is a well developed and somewhat undernourished man lying
quietly in bed in no distress. He is mentally clear.

Skull--Symmetrical. No exostoses. irregularities or tenderness.
Scalp--Is clean and there are no scars. Hair--Grey, fair in amount and fine
in texture. Face--The patient appears younger than he is in reality. Skin--Is
pale with a definite yellow lemon color tinge. It is smooth, warm and
moderately dry. There are no eruptions, scaling or pigmentation. Eyes--The
pupils are round and equal. The sclerae are yellowish blue. No photophobia,
lacrimation, diplopia, nystagmus, palsies, lid-lag or exophthalmos. The
                                                              of the right eye.
conjunctivae are clear and there are no gross disturbances of vision. The
vision of the left eye is less than that of the right due to previous injury.
Ears--No discharge, stigmata, or tophi. Nose--No deformities, obstruction or
discharge. Mouth--The breath is odorless. No ulcerations, exudate or pigmentation
Lips--Normal in color. No herpes, ulcerations or fissures. Teeth--Numerous
missing. Many fillings. Gums--Reddish pale. No pyorrhoea, bleeding or leadline
tongue--Is red and smooth and fissured. No tremor or mucous patches. Tonsils--
Not enlarged and there is no exudate. Pharynx--Pale. No catarrh. Reflexes
present. Larynx--The voice is not remarkable. Neck--The thyroid is not
palpable. No bruits, thrills, pulsations, stiffness or tracheal tug. Lymph
glands not enlarged

C. E.   Symmetrical. Expansion is equal on both sides. Respirations not
accelerated or shallow. No abnormal pulsations.

H. E.   The apex impulse is felt 10 cm from the midsternal line in the

5.

PETER BENT BRIGHAM HOSPITAL
MEDICAL SERVICE
NAME   WARD   F-2   MED. NO.

the nipple line. By percussion the L.B.D. is 10 cm. R.B.D. is . cm. The
supracardiac dulness is 4 cm. On auscultation no bruits or thrills are heard.

Aorta   To percussion the supracardiac dulness is . cm. Palpation and auscultatic
do not reveal any bruits or thrills

Peripheral Vessels—Arteries—The radial pulses are synchronous, regular in rhythm and
in rate. No arteriolsclaerosis.

Veins—No abnormalities noted

Blood Pressure   Systolic 90   Diastolic 40

Lungs   Resonant thrdout. Breath sounds are vesicular and no rales are heard.
Tactile fremitus is not increased or decreased. Lower borders move well

Abdomen   Is well developed and symmetrical. No pulsations or peristalsis,
tenderness, masses or spasm. No hernia or fluid. Reflexes are present.

Liver   Not palpable.

Gall Bladder, Spleen, Kidneys, Bladder—Not palpable

Genitalia   Hernial rings not enlarged.

Lymphatic Glands —Not enlarged in the neck, axillae, or epitrochlear regions. There
are a few glands in the groins

Bones   Spine shows no scoliosis, lordosis, rigidity or tenderness. Other bones
not remarkable

Extremities   Arms—Show no involuntary movements, wasting, tremor or clubbed fingers
Nails not remarkable. Biceps, triceps and radial periosteal reflexes present
No joint changes.

Legs—Show no varicosities, scars or ulcers. Knee jerks slightly
exaggerated. Achilles and plantar reflexes present. Babinski and Oppenheim
negative. No edema or joint changes. Ankle clonus negative. Kernig and
Romberg negative.

Sensation   No anesthesia, paresthesia, or hyperesthesia.

History   The patient is a single Nova Scotian machinist aged 46 who is admitted
to the hospital for the first time complaining of weakness and shortness of breath

P. I. began about 20 months ago, in June 1924 with a sensation of
distress in the region of the stomach and in the lower part of the abdomen
which came usually after meals. This was soon followed by loss of appetite,
intense soreness of the tongue and weakness. Five months after the onset of the
disease, due to weakness, he was forced to give up his job. Nine months after

Chart continued on the following page

-6-

PETER BENT BRIGHAM HOSPITAL
MEDICAL SERVICE

NAME   WARD   P_&_MED. NO.

the onset of the illness, in Feb. 1925, his condition began to improve and in
June 1925 he was well to such a degree as to be able to resume his work. One
month later, however, the symptoms of weakness returned and since that time
he has grown worse. About two months before admission to the hospital he noticed
shortness of breath on slight exertion, failing vision and numbness of the fingers
and toes.

On physical examination he is/poorly nourished, his skin is lemon
yellow in color and his tongue is red and smooth. The examination of other
organs is negative

Diagnosis   Pernicious Anaemia

(?) Subacute Combined Degeneration of the Cord

(Dr. Herrmann)
(Dr. Fried)

Jan. 15.   (Dr. Sturgis) - The patient has the typical appearance, history and
blood findings of pernicious anemia. The papillae of the tongue are very atrophied.
Skin has a definitely yellow tint.

(Dr. Sturgis)
(per L.V.M.)

Jan. 17.   This patient entered the hospital 4 days ago, with a normal
temperature, pulse rate, and respirations. His clinical pathology showed a
hemoglobin of 13% Dare, red blood count of 756,000; white blood count of 2,600
with a differential count of 72% polymorphonuclears, and a smear which was
typical of primary anemia. Admission specimen of urine was entirely negative.
Two stool examinations showed a double plus benzidine, but a negative urine
reaction. Blood serum reaction on January 15th was negative. Repeat count
one on the following day showed a red count of 895,000; fractional gastric
analysis showed no free hydrochloric acid. In spite of his rather marked
anemia, he showed no signs of anoxemia, so I think it would be much better to
wait for a few days to see if his count will rise rapidly. If his count
continues to fall, transfusion will be done immediately. The diagnosis of
pernicious anemia, seems very certain, so the patient will be turned over to
r. Murphy and r. Monroe, for detailed study of his blood condition.

(Dr. Herrmann)

-7-

PETER BENT BRIGHAM HOSPITAL
MEDICAL SERVICE

NAME   WARD   2nd   MED. NO

Jan.17.   Blood Pressure - Systolic 105; diastolic 70.   (Dr. Falk)

Jan.   .   (Dr. MacPherson) - There is slight diminution in recognition
of light touch in the fingers and toes. Vibratory sense impaired in the
left leg. No definite evidence of injury to the cortico-spinal tracts.

(Dr. MacPherson)
(per L.B.H.)

Jan.   .   On January the 15th this patient also had a sudden rise in
fever to 100.8° with no rise in pulse rate or respirations. Physical
examination at this time showed acute upper respiratory infection,
with pharyngitis and some coryza. No other evidence of inflammation could
be found, which could be considered as the cause of this fever. Since that
time the cold has persisted and he has had slight rises in fever, until
yesterday. There has been moderate improvement in his clinical appearance,
and one count done on January 17th, showed almost a doubling of his admission
count. The count repeated however, on January 20th, showed 760,000 which
was a slight gain over his admission count.   Because of his rather low
count it seemed advisable to group his blood and it was found to be group IV.
Bile index on admission was 15, and done on January 20th, was 10.
After a few more days study he will be put on a high purin diet, to see if there
will be any effect on the rapidity of regeneration of his white blood count.

(Dr. Herrmann)

Jan.31.   During the past week, this patient has been very much upset
because of his lack of appetite, inability to take the high purin diet.
It has been observed that until these patients show a definite improvement
in the blood condition it is very difficult for them to take the diet, and
it is very easy for them to become discouraged, and willing to drop it all.
This man apparently has been in that frame of mind during the past week,
and Dr. Murphy and I have talked over the whole situation with him, and I am
sure that he has realized his mistake of wanting to go home immediately. On
January 26th, this patient had a very sudden but definite diarrhoea, which
caused him a great deal of discomfort. Contrary to the old ideas/reservations
made on the new patients we have been treating with high purin diet, the
diarrhoea, usually precedes the marked rise in the blood count. Following this
diarrhoea, on the following day, the white count was 900,000. It is very
interesting to see if there is any appreciable rise during the coming week.

Chart continued on the following page

-8-

PETER BENT BRIGHAM HOSPITAL
MEDICAL SERVICE

NAME   WARD   MED. NO

The question of transfusion has been brought up, and if the patient does not react quickly to the purin diet, he will be given a transfusion, and then will be put back on the high purin diet. Further studies are being made at the present time.

(Dr. Herrmann)

Feb.4.   Ophthalmoscopic examination:-   The retinae and discs are markedly paler than the average. There are no areas of hemorrhages or exudate. Venous pulsations are seen in both eyes. The arteries are of normal caliber and tortuosity and do not produce any nicking at the arteriovenous crossings. The veins are not engorged. The media are clear.

(Dr. Falk)

Feb.7.   During the past week, there has been a remarkable change in this patient's condition, and his attitude towards his diet. At the present time he takes the high purine diet with great ease. His count on January 29th was 1,000,000. Following this there was a very marked sudden rise in his reticulated red count, and 1.6% to 15.5% and a corresponding sudden rise in his red count from 1,000,000 to 2,760,000. Associated with this marked rise in red count there has been a corresponding improvement in his general condition, and at the present time he has lost all his former feeling of weakness, and dissatisfaction. This patient seems to have been a very good test for the high purin diet and I am of the opinion that the dietary regulations is directly responsible for this remission. It is hard to conceive that the remissions brought about in cases of primary anemia, treated with this diet have been coincidental with the diet, and not directly responsible to it. He is being closely followed by Dr. Monroe, and Dr. Murphy.

(Dr. Herrmann)

Feb.14.   This patient has continued to make rapid progress in his blood condition on the high purine diet, and his red blood count is now above 3,000,000, and he will be allowed to be up and about the ward in preparation for discharge. Symptomatically he is greatly improved, cooperative, and has gained 2.2 kilograms in weight during the past week.

(Dr. Falk)

-9-

PETER BENT BRIGHAM HOSPITAL
MEDICAL SERVICE

NAME   WARD   2nd. MED NO

In view of the fact that the patient's condition was steadily improving it was decided that he was fit to be discharged home. During the past week, he has done very well, but has had no complaints. A repeated test meal was done by Dr. Lasser which failed to show any free hydrochloric acid. He will be followed by Dr. Murphy, and will continue his special diet.

Discharged to Dr. Murphy.

Result - improved.

(Dr. Falk)

Chart continued on the following page

PETER BENT BRIGHAM HOSPITAL

MEDICAL SERVICE

NAME　　　　　　　　　　　　　　　　　　　WARD F-2nd.　MED. NO.

Jan.15.　　　Wassermann reaction:- (blood serum) negative.　(Miss Underhill)

Jan.17.　　　Gastric analysis:-　Fasting specimen Specimen I

Vol 30 c.c. white, watery, no gross blood or pus.　Slight amount of mucus.

Microscopic examination:- Moderate W.B.C., No R.B.C., Sarcinae, or Oppler-Boas bacilli.　Benzidine - negative. Free Acid - 0. Combined - 8. Total acidity - 8.　　　　　　　　　　　　(Dr. Falk)

Jan.17.　　　Test meal - Specimen II

No specimen.

Specimen III - 60 minutes after test meal.

10 c.c. white 5% food particles.　Free acid - 0. Combined 7. Total acidity - 7.

Specimen IV. 120 minutes after test meal was given.

10 c.c., white 5% food particles.　Free Acid - 0. Combined - 5. Total acidity - 5.　　　　　　　　　(Dr. Falk)

Feb.21.　　　Test meal.

A. Fasting specimen.
1. vol 20 c.c.
2. Free HCl - 0.
3. Combined Hcl - 5.

B. one hour after test meal.
1. Vol 5 c.c.
2. Free HCl - 0.
3. Combined HCl - 10.

(Dr. Massee)

Jan.14.　　　Stool - formed, brown, benzidine - ++ Guiac - 0. Neutral. No starch, fat, meat fibres, mucus, pus, ova or parasites.

Jan.15.　　　Bile index 15　　　　　　　　(Dr. Murphy

Jan.20.　　　Blood grouping group IV　　　(Miss Adkinson)

Jan.20.　　　Bile index - 10.　　　　　　(Dr. Murphy)

Jan.20　　　Stool - formed, brown, benzidine - ++ Guiac - +

Feb.2.　　　Bile index - 8.　　　　　　(Dr. Murphy)

Feb.9.　　　Blood uric acid 4.2 mgms. per 100 c.c.

Feb.9　　　Bile index 5.　　　　　　(Dr. Murphy)

PETER BENT BRIGHAM HOSPITAL
MEDICAL SERVICE

URINE

NAME   WARD P-2nd MED. NO.

Date	Color	Reaction	Sp. Gr.	Albumen	Sugar	
Jan. 14.	Clear amber	neut.	1020	0	0	Sediment:- No W.B.C., R.B.C., or casts.
Jan. 15.	Clear amber	neut.	1012	0	0	Sediment:- 1700 c.c. No W.B.C., R.B.C., or casts
Jan. 27.	Clear amber	acid	1015	0	0	Sediment:- No W.B.C., R.B.C., or casts.
Feb. 6.	Hazy straw	acid	1065	0	0	Sediment:- Rare W.B.C., No R.B.C., or casts.
Feb. 15.	Hazy amber	acid	1032	0	0	Sediment:- Numerous W.B.C., No R.B.C., or casts.

BLOOD

Date	
Jan. 14	Hemoglobin 13% Dare, R.B.C. 775,000. W.B.C. 3,600. Smear:- polymorphonuclears 72%; lymphocytes 18%; large mononuclears 8%; eosinophiles 2%. Marked poikilocytosis, and anisocytosis. Slight diffuse basophilia. Slight polychromatophilia. Three nucleated R.B.C. Platelets normal. Reticulated R.B.C. 0.7% 2000 cells.
Jan. 15.	R.B.C. 750,000.
Jan. 15.	Hemoglobin 13% Dare. R.B.C. 895,000
Jan. 15.	Hemoglobin 15% S. R.B.C. 875,000.
Jan. 16.	Venepuncture count reticulated R.B.C. 0.7% 2000 cells (Dr. Monroe)
Jan. 17.	Hemoglobin 16% S. R.B.C. 1,370,000. Reticulated R.B.C. 0.8% 2000cells
Jan. 20.	Hemoglobin 20% S. R.B.C. 860,000. Reticulated R.B.C. 0.3%

Chart continued on the following page

PETER BENT BRIGHAM HOSPITAL
MEDICAL SERVICE

URINE

NAME _____   WARD F-2nd.   MED. NO.

Date	Color	Reaction	Sp. Gr.	Albumen	Sugar	
			.			

BLOOD

Date	
Jan.23.	Hemoglobin 17% S. R.B.C. 875,000. Reticulated R.B.C. 0.4%
Jan.27.	Hemoglobin 18% S. R.B.C. 900,000. W.B.C. 3,450. Reticulated R.B.C. 0.3%
Jan.29.	Hemoglobin 20% S. R.B.C. 1,050,000. Reticulated R.B.C. 1.6%
Jan.31.	R.B.C. 1,150. Reticulated R.B.C. 5,6%. Smear:- polymorphonuclears 48%; lymphocytes 39%; large mononuclears 10%; eosinophiles 3%. Marked polychromatophilia. Nucleated R.B.C. 0.2%
Feb.2.	Hemoglobin 23% S. R.B.C. 1,560,000. Reticulated R.B.C. 15.5%
Feb.4.	Hemoglobin 33% S. R.B.C. 1,970,000. Reticulated R.B.C. 0.8% 2000 cells
Feb.6.	Hemoglobin 35% S. R.B.C. 2,760,000. Reticulated R.B.C. 3.6% - 2000 cells
Feb.9.	Hemoglobin 46% S. R.B.C. 2,740,000. W.B.C. 4,650. Reticulated R.B.C. 2.3% - 2000 cells.
Feb.14.	Hemoglobin 61% S. R.B.C. 3,700,000. Reticulated R.B.C. 0.5%

According to Sturgis,[387] the first public mention that liver might benefit patients with pernicious anemia was made by Minot at a meeting of the Suffolk District Medical Society in Boston on April 28, 1926. Along with other physicians of the staff of the Collis P. Huntington Memorial Hospital of Boston, Minot participated in discussing the various phases of malignant lymphoma at that meeting. Minot stated[387] that "toward the end of my speech I had a little something to say about pernicious anemia and in the course of not over three minutes I told them that I thought patients with pernicious anemia might be greatly benefited by feeding them liver generously." Apparently, no publication covered the remarks of the evening, and no particular enthusiasm was aroused in the audience by Minot's statement.[387]

In May 1926, Minot and Murphy[297] reported to the Association of American Physicians their observations on patients with pernicious anemia partaking of a special diet. Although this report was the first public announcement of the demonstrated efficacy of liver therapy in pernicious anemia, it was not published until subsequent to the report that appeared in the *Journal of the American Medical Association* in October 1926.[298]

The details of this special diet were reported by Murphy and Minot in the *Boston Medical and Surgical Journal* in 1926,[303] and in October 1926, Minot and Murphy[298] published their dramatic report of

Average Red Blood Corpuscle Count *

Before Diet Started		After Diet Started					
		About 1 Month		About 2 Months		4 to 6 Months	
Number of Cases	Average R. B. C. Count in Millions	Number of Cases	Average R. B. C. Count in Millions	Number of Cases†	Average R. B. C. Count in Millions	Number of Cases†	Average R. B. C. Count in Millions
19	0.90	19	3.28	15	4.08	12	4.50
15	1.60	15	3.25	13	4.09	10	4.54
11	2.30	11	3.83	9	4.41	5	4.47
45	1.47	45	3.40	37	4.16	27	4.50

* The figures represent the count per cubic millimeter before and after starting special diet in three groups of cases of pernicious anemia: (1) with less than 1.2 million; (2) having from 1.2 to 2 million, and (3) having from 2 to 2.75 million before diet was begun. Also, averages for all forty-five cases are shown.
† The differences in the number of cases after about one month is because some have not taken the diet for as long as two, and others as long as four months.

Figure 31. Figure from Minot and Murphy's 1926 publication demonstrating the efficacy of liver therapy in pernicious anemia. (From J. Amer. Med. Ass. 87:470, 1926. © 1926 by the American Medical Association.)

the "treatment of pernicious anemia by a special diet." Forty-five
patients with pernicious anemia were fed a diet of 120 to 240 grams of
cooked calf or beef liver and 120 grams or more of beef or mutton
muscle meat. Clinical improvement was "heralded in the peripheral
blood before the end of the first week by the beginning of a most
definite rise of the reticulocytes (young red blood corpuscles) of from
about 1.0 percent to usually about 8.0 and even 15.5 percent of all the
red blood cells. . . . By the end of the second week, these cells usually
had returned close to their normal percentage." Figures 31 and 32
reproduced from Minot and Murphy's original paper[298] demonstrate
the hematological improvement after the administration of liver. As a
tribute to their epochal contributions, Minot, Murphy, and Whipple[300,304,428] were awarded the Nobel Prize in Physiology and Medicine
in 1934 (Fig. 33).

In 1927, one year after the discovery of liver therapy for pernicious
anemia, Peabody[321] demonstrated that after treatment with liver, the
bone marrow of patients with pernicious anemia converted from megaloblastic to normoblastic type erythropoiesis. In 1928, Cohn et al.[94]
studied the properties of the material in liver that was effective in
producing a hematological remission in patients with pernicious
anemia. They determined that the active principle was water soluble,
ether soluble, and precipitated by ethanol. It was found in the filtrate

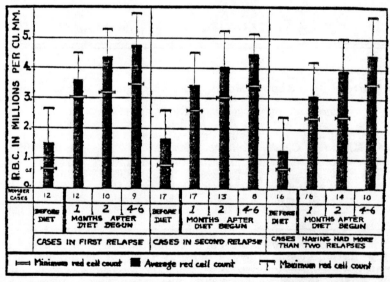

Red blood cell counts in forty-five cases of pernicious anemia before and after beginning special diet. Cases grouped according to the number of relapses the patients
had had. One and two months after diet began indicates an approximate amount of
time and for any given case is not less and often somewhat more than four or eight
weeks. The differences in the total number of cases after about one month are caused
by the fact that some patients have had the diet for less than two, and others for less
than four, months.

Figure 32.   Figure from Minot and Murphy's 1926 publication. (From J. Amer. Med.
Ass. 87:470, 1926. © 1926 by the American Medical Association.)

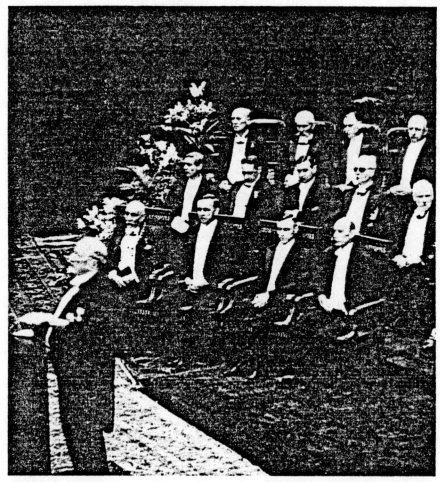

Figure 33. The Nobel ceremonies of December 10, 1934. In the front row seated on the far left is Italian playwright Luigi Pirandello, Nobel Laureate in Literature, followed by Whipple, Murphy, and Minot receiving the Nobel Prize in Physiology and Medicine. (Reproduced with permission of William P. Murphy, M.D.)

from basic lead acetate and was precipitable by phosphotungstic acid. As a result of their studies, Cohn et al.[94] developed a potent aqueous extract of liver that could be given parenterally to patients with pernicious anemia. At the time it was also reported that the anemia resulting from *D. latum* infestation closely resembled pernicious anemia and could be corrected with liver therapy.[37,359]

Prior to 1929, the diagnosis of pernicious anemia during life was made primarily on the basis of peripheral blood findings. Although megaloblasts were sometimes observed in the blood and served as important diagnostic indicators of pernicious anemia, megaloblasts in the bone marrow were usually observed only in necropsy material. Mikhail Arinkin (Fig. 34) in 1929[17] was the first to develop and

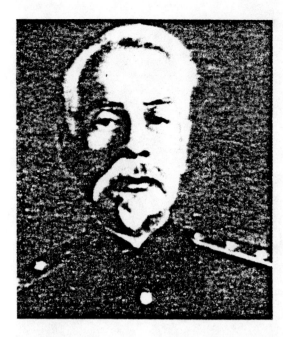

Figure 34. Mikhail Innoken-
tevich Arinkin (1876-1948).
From Problems of Hematology
and Blood Transfusion 4:72,
1959. Reproduced with permission of Pergamon Press, Oxford,
England.)

popularize the technique of sternal bone marrow aspiration during
life. His technique made it possible, for the first time in the history of
pernicious anemia, to view megaloblastic changes in the bone marrow
during life. Arinkin's contribution was a significant advance for perni-

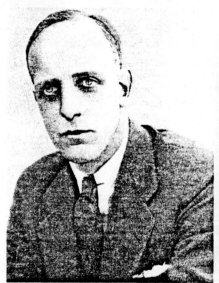 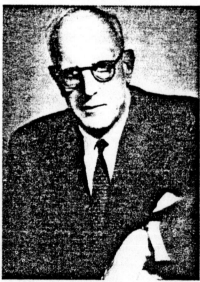

Figure 35. Left: William B. Castle in 1932 as associate professor of medicine at Harvard Medical School and Associate Director, Thorndike Memorial Laboratory. (Courtesy of William B. Castle, M.D.) Right: William B. Castle (1897-   ). (From Medicine
43:617, 1964. © 1964 by The Williams & Wilkins Co., Baltimore, Md.)

cious anemia as well as for other hematological disorders and enabled the diagnosis of megaloblastic anemia to be made with greater assurance than was possible when peripheral blood abnormalities were the only diagnostic criteria available.

Following closely upon the empirical observations of Minot and Murphy,[297,298] Castle and Locke[78] in 1928 published a short abstract in the *Journal of Clinical Investigation* entitled "Observations on the etiological relationship of achylia gastrica to pernicious anemia." William B. Castle (Fig. 35) recalled the generation of the ideas leading to his pioneering investigations:[384]

> The "idea" of a functional relationship between defective gastric digestion and pernicious anemia happened to formulate itself in terms of an experimental approach at a particular moment in 1927. Of course, all the necessary data had been known to me for some months or even for years, such as the nearly universal incidence of achylia gastrica.
>
> Nevertheless, I recall very clearly that sometime early in 1927, I was leaving the Thorndike to go across town to a meeting of the American Academy of Arts and Sciences, at which Dr. Minot was to speak about the present state of his work with liver extracts. My lease of life at the Thorndike, having been generously extended during that year by Francis Peabody and Joe Wearn on the basis of no tangible accomplishment on my part, caused me to feel some urge to make a favorable impression on Dr. Minot, some of whose liver fractions we were testing at the Thorndike. At any rate, I left the laboratory on the fourth floor of the Thorndike, that you will remember, without any specific plan in mind. However, while descending in the "back elevator" the idea of digesting beef steak in the human stomach and administering it subsequent to a control period of beef muscle alone, did occur to me. The reticulocyte response that we were using in the evaluation of liver extracts meant that a "yes or no" answer could be obtained in 20 days, only the last 10 of which would involve any personal inconvenience. After Dr. Minot's lecture I talked with him informally and described to him, creating the impression, I hoped, of a carefully thought out experimental design, the thought that had suddenly penetrated a slow-moving mind only an hour or two previously. He was, as usual, at once interested in a new idea, irrespective of its source. Our observations began in February, 1927. They were first reported in May, 1928, to the Young Turks. I sat up all night in Boston preparing my ten minute talk and saw the dawn. While shaving, I noticed that my hair had turned grey at the temples.*

In the published abstract of this talk, Castle and Locke[78] reported that the stomach content of a normal man after one hour following a meal of 300 grams of rare hamburger given to pernicious anemia patients daily caused a reticulocyte response in eight of ten patients. Administration of hamburger with pernicious anemia gastric juice or crude pig gastric mucous membrane did not cause this type of response. The authors concluded that "the normal gastric mucosa alone, or through their action on food proteins, can produce some substances capable on oral administration of definitely benefiting certain cases of pernicious anemia."

In the first full length account of these investigations, Castle[79] in 1929 investigated the effect of the administration to patients with per-

---

*Reprinted, with permission, from Strauss, M. B. Of medicine, men and molecules. Medicine 43:619, 1964. © 1964, The Williams & Wilkins Co., Baltimore.

nicious anemia of the contents of the normal human stomach recovered after the ingestion of beef muscle. In eight of these ten patients fed with the gastric contents of a normal man recovered 45 minutes to one hour after a meal of 300 grams of rare beef muscle, increased numbers of reticulocytes and hematological improvement resulted. Castle concluded that "there is found in the normal stomach during the digestion of beef muscle some substance capable of promptly and markedly relieving the anemia of these patients." He stated that the recovery was due to either a direct action of the same constituents of the secretions produced by the normal man or some action of these secretions on the meat. Beef muscle alone fed to the pernicious anemia patients did not have an effect on the blood.

In this and subsequent reports, Castle et al.[80-83] determined that an "intrinsic factor" was present in the gastric secretions of normal persons but absent from the gastric juice of pernicious anemia patients. Their studies provided the solid link for the long-suspected relationship between achylia gastrica and pernicious anemia. Presumably Castle's "extrinsic factor" or dietary factor found in meats was the yet-to-be isolated vitamin B_{12}. Castle's initial findings led to almost immediate therapeutic applications, for in 1929 Sturgis and Isaacs[386] reported that the oral administration of desiccated hog stomach could lead to a hematological remission in untreated pernicious anemia patients. Apparently, the hog stomach was a source of exogenous intrinsic factor.

Events leading to the isolation and crystallization of vitamin B_{12} in 1948[345,375] had their beginning in the production of an aqueous extract of liver by Cohn et al.[94] in 1928. This extract was highly potent and could be given parenterally, thereby possessing some advantages over the large amounts of liver needed for oral liver therapy. Although effective, the parenteral extract often varied in potency and occasionally caused serious allergic reactions.

Observations that microbial substances could exhibit vitamin activity and produce hematological remissions in macrocytic anemias were made during the 1930s. Although the hematopoietically active substances produced by these microorganisms were probably folates, these studies were among the first to suggest that microbial systems could be used in the investigation of antianemic substances. Wills and Evans[437] in 1938 demonstrated that a "new" hematopoietic factor found in autolyzed yeast extracts could produce a reticulocytosis in tropical macrocytic anemia, and in 1939, Wintrobe[438] found that dehydrated brewer's yeast produced a hematopoietic response in five pernicious anemia patients.

In addition to the original aqueous liver extract isolated by Cohn et al. in 1928[94] and the observations of Wills and Evans[437] and Wintrobe[438] that hematopoietic activity was associated with microbial substances, other factors leading to the isolation and crystallization of vitamin B_{12} began to appear. Some of these had their origin in agricultural and animal husbandry studies. In 1944, Martin[284] found that ruminant animals feeding on pastures deficient in cobalt developed anemia and that this type of anemia could be cured or prevented by administration of cobalt. Later in 1947, Mary Shorb,[370] in the Department of Poultry Husbandry at the University of Maryland, studied certain growth factors necessary for chicken nutrition. She discovered that an "unidentified growth factor" contained in commercial liver extracts used to treat pernicious anemia was required for the growth of *Lactobacillus lactis* Dorner in an amino acid basal medium containing all the synthetic B vitamins. In her report, Shorb postulated that this "growth factor" might be the "active principle in pernicious anemia."

Meanwhile, intensive efforts to isolate the active principle from liver extracts had been in progress for some time on both sides of the Atlantic. At Merck and Co. in the U.S.A., Karl Folkers headed the group of investigators involved in these efforts. Folkers quickly and astutely recognized that Shorb's microbiological technique might expedite the efforts of the Merck team to isolate the active principle from liver for several reasons. First, her microbial method provided a convenient bioassay system for antipernicious anemia substances. Second, and of special importance, it circumvented the need for untreated pernicious anemia patients as assay systems for these substances.

Recently, Karl Folkers, currently Director of the Institute for Biomedical Research at the University of Texas at Austin, related to the author some of his recollections regarding his key role in the dramatic events leading up to and surrounding the isolation of crystalline vitamin B_{12} by the Merck team in 1948:

During my three years as a Post-Doctorate at Yale University, Treat Baldwin Johnson was my Professor. "T.B." completely changed my professional preferences from organic chemistry and physical chemistry to a strong medical orientation. He rarely gave me chemical journals with articles which he thought I should read, but he frequently gave me issues of the *Journal of the American Medical Association,* which contained feature articles on chemistry and medicine. Our frequent discussions were generally on reactions to synthesize new compounds of potential medical interest. "T.B.'s" visions for chemistry and medicine were "ahead of his time." Based on such inspirations, my career has ever since been medically oriented. . . .

When I was offered two industrial positions in 1934, "T.B." pointed out that I might accept the offer from Merck and Co. Inc. in New Jersey to join their newly formed Laboratory of Pure Research. This Laboratory offered opportunities which both "T.B." and I recognized to do basic chemical research to benefit medicine. . . .
At Yale, "T.B." and I had monitored publications from Germany on the vitamin we know today as thiamin, and I had begun to perceive that if one were to elucidate the chemical structures of new vitamins, one had first to solve their isolation in pure form.

During my personnel interviews at Merck, Dr. Randolph Major asked me what I was interested in, and listened patiently to my discussion of the literature on the vitamin of unknown structure (thiamin). Although he recounted the remarks of his peers that vitamins offered academic but little commercial interest, I nevertheless accepted his offer to do pure research in his laboratory.

Dr. Major initially assigned alkaloid problems to me, but in four years, he appointed me Assistant Director of Research and I suddenly became responsible for determining the structure and for synthesizing vitamin B_6, which had just been isolated there in the laboratories of Dr. John Keresztesy.

Dr. Stanton Harris, Dr. Eric Stiller and I achieved a "scientific-first" on the structure of vitamin B_6 in 1939, and Stan and I published the first synthesis of vitamin B_6 the same year. Only a few days after we had found that the synthetic vitamin B_6 hydrochloride and the natural specimen were identical, Dr. Major asked a question like, "What are you going to do next?" I remember being momentarily angry about that question, because Stan and I had worked very intensely for a year or so, and had even neglected our vacations. After I had "recharged my battery," I realized that Dr. Major had asked a sound and reasonable question. . . . Initiated by vitamin B_6, Eric Stiller, Stan Harris, Jake Finkelstein, John Keresztesy and I solved and published the total synthesis of pure pantothenic acid in 1940. . . . and independently, Stan Harris, Don Wolf, Ralph Mozingo, and I at Merck achieved the synthesis and stereochemistry of biotin during 1943-1945. We had barely achieved synthetic biotin, when we undertook the war-time and urgent isolation of pure penicillin and achieved the pure antibiotic.

These years of research on isolations, including vitamin B_6 and biotin, were important to the subsequent discovery of vitamin B_{12}, because we had learned by hard experience how to isolate natural products and understood such risky, very difficult, and very time-consuming tasks. I had personally started by relatively easy isolations of alkaloids. Then, through associations as Assistant Director, particularly with John Keresztesy, I became realistic on the challenge and the hardship of the isolation of an unknown vitamin which is far more difficult than the isolation of an alkaloid or an antibiotic. In those days, the isolation of an unknown vitamin was described like, "finding a needle in a haystack."

I had become intellectually prepared for difficult isolations by bioassays to guide chemical fractionations. In reviewing the literature on "Unidentified Vitamins" to make an invited presentation at a Conference on "The Chemistry and Physiology of Growth" in celebration of the Bi-Centennial of Princeton University in 1946, I said:

"Now that the chemistry of pteroylglutamic acid and its related conjugates is known, it is likely that more rapid progress will be made in the isolation of the liver antipernicious anemia factor(s). The unknown factor or factors for pernicious anemia in liver and other sources are possibly the outstanding unidentified factors of today, if importance is judged by the amount of clinical evidence on therapeutic usefulness." (p. 81, Princeton University Press, 1949.)

In discussing my proposed research with Dr. Major to isolate the antipernicious anemia factor, he was unimpressed, and his response was something like, "Who are you—to think that you could solve that problem where others have failed for so long!" He explained that he and Dr. Hans Molitor had considered this project, but had given up the idea, and they had received no encouragement from their outside medical advisors. However, Dr. Major was a flexible Director. He said he would discuss my proposal with the well-known biochemist, Dr. Henry Dakin, who at that time was a member of the Merck Board of Directors. Dr. Dakin was a perceptive man of considerable wisdom, and . . . his response to Dr. Major was something like, "Of course, let Karl have a go at it"—and, "I shall send him a bottle of one of my initial liver fractions."

Dr. Major had sent me to an annual meeting of a medical society in Atlantic City. He frequently encouraged me to attend both chemical and medical meetings. I met Randolph West, M.D., in the lobby of the Claridge Hotel. We slightly knew each other, and he asked me what I was doing. To my comment that I wanted to work on the isolation of the antipernicious anemia factor, and to try chromatography to achieve further purification, he asked, "What is chromatography?" He offered no judgment on my reply, but promptly said he would test my fractions, and then explained how few patients with pernicious anemia would be available even in the metropolitan area of New York. He was on the faculty in Hematology at the College of Physicians and Surgeons of Columbia University.

I reported to Dr. Major that I had fortuitously met Dr. West who volunteered to test my fractions from the chromatographic experiments of the crude liver residue to be provided to me by Dr. Dakin. Dr. Major was satisfied.

I and an assistant, Frank Koniuszy, dissolved a little of the blackish liver residue in an aqueous medium and passed the solution over a column of alumina as judged to be the right way to go about such chromatography on the basis of our limited experience on isolating alkaloids. The eluate from the column was colorless, because the black "junk" of the liver residue had stuck to the top of the column. Fearing that the antipernicious anemia factor might not be too stable, we lyophilized the eluate to obtain a white residue. An aliquot was mailed to Dr. West to test on the first available patient. Dr. West looked at the white sample and immediately called Dr. Dakin, to whom he said something like, "My God, Folkers has already crystallized the antipernicious anemia factor." Such a pronouncement caused Dr. Dakin to telephone immediately Dr. Major to ask for a report. Dr. Major replied that he knew nothing about it, but would get a report from me. Within minutes, I was called to his office and asked to explain why I hadn't informed him that I had crystallized the factor. My response was something like "Who, me?—I haven't done any such thing!" Then I remembered having seen the white ice pattern of the lyophilized residue, and explained that this appearance of a crystalline structure had been mistakenly viewed by Dr. West as the "crystalline factor." Obviously, Dr. West tested such a remarkable sample and, indeed, found that it was active in causing remission of the anemia.

Chromatography was not common then. Today, it is routine. That first chromatographic experiment and its emotional impact were truly momentous. I realized that the active factor had successfully passed through a column of alumina, and that this result was not to be expected were the factor protein-like as could be implied from the literature. So, the factor was probably not a peptide or protein, and it appeared certain that it could be purified by chromatography. Randolph West wanted more fractions to test and Dr. Dakin and Dr. Major were more enthusiastic, as was I.

I went to Chicago, and to the dismay of the Accounting Department, arranged for crude liver extracts, equivalent to tons of liver. We fractionated, and Dr. West established a network in New York to find pernicious anemia patients for tests. Over a period of time, we learned some basic facts about the chemical nature of the antipernicious anemia factor which were of considerable importance and solely by the hematological responses of Dr. West's anemia patients. We learned that chromatography by various procedures was really successful, and that the factor was relatively stable, and that it could be distributed between certain solvents, and that it could be of relatively low molecular weight, and that it surely was not a peptide or protein . . . I was continuously and acutely aware of the need to discern a chemical or physical property which could correlate with activity and minimize the need for clinical tests. We had many positive fractions by Dr. West's tests and a few inactive ones, and were really not very far from the end although we didn't know it. . . .

One day, I took a trip to the University of Maryland to visit Dr. George Briggs, and to discuss a possible project involving pantothenic acid. I asked George about the regulatory conditions the University of Maryland would expect Merck to satisfy if we were to work together.

Dr. Briggs took a rejected proposal from his desk which he said would illustrate the contractual conditions of the University for cooperation with an industry. The proposal had been written by Dr. Mary Shorb and was based on her very limited microbiological data with *L. lactis* Dorner with crude liver extracts which were available for the treatment of pernicious anemia. The proposal was to seek financial support to continue her microbiological study, and the proposal had been declined by two prominent pharmaceutical companies and one foundation. Interestingly, these two companies and the foundation had an actual research basis to be very interested in the significance of her proposal. Their declinations could be considered due to errors of judgment. Her data were so limited and it was too incredible at that time that there could be any relationship between the growth of an organism on crude liver extracts and the hematological response of a patient with pernicious anemia to the same extracts. Dr. Shorb's financial need was actually very modest . . . .

I explained to George Briggs and Mary Shorb what I was doing about the antipernicious anemia factor, and that I would like to give her data the benefit of the doubt, and to see if a spectrum of our positive and negative liver fractions from the tests on patients with pernicious anemia would show any correlation with the growth of *L. lactis* Dorner. We did not pursue the project involving pantothenic acid which had been the sole basis for my visit there!

I realized on the way home that those at Merck who acted on outside grants could also be negative. Consequently, I saw Dr. Major early the next morning, recounted my visit to Maryland, and asked for his approval of a sum so small, that he might immediately say "yes" to my desire to finance assays on our fractions for a few months by Mary Shorb. I explained that I could readily tell if there were a promising correlation between the growth of her microorganism and the response of the human disease to our fractions. Both he and I readily visualized the great significance of the potential correlation. True to his openmindedness and understanding, he replied, "Yes."

Dr. Shorb's assay significantly expedited the final steps of isolation, and particularly made possible the search for vitamin B_{12} in fermentation materials as a practical source for commercialization. This search culminated on the day that Ed Rickes spotted some beautiful red crystals growing out of a blood-red solution which was derived from a fermentation broth. The crystalline vitamin was achieved both from liver and the fermentation source only a few days apart. The exceptional judgment and experimental skill of Dr. Norman Brink, who finalized the crystallization of vitamin B_{12} from liver fractions, more than matched their paucity and high financial value.

The first clinical test of the crystalline vitamin was indeed an emotional highlight. Norm Brink had made a solution of a few micrograms of the crystals for injections by Dr. West to three patients, and he then lyophilized the aliquots. When he showed me the ampoules, I remarked that one could see nothing, because a few micrograms of the substance per ampoule was almost invisible to the unaided eye. I had some doubt about how Dr. West would respond to an "empty ampoule," and asked Norm to put some saline in the ampoule so that there would be "something" for Dr. West to see. Also, we made up a table of data for Dr. West to justify our recommendation that he administer dosages as small as 3, 6 and 150 μg to three patients.

This time, I could say to Dr. West that I thought we really had the pure factor. This situation was in contrast to the time of the first sample that he had received. The right number of days later, he called me at home to describe the very strong and prompt hematopoietic response. We had succeeded.

Several months before the day of the crystalline vitamin, I had been in Zurich, Switzerland, sitting in the garden of the Baur au Lac Hotel reading mail from the lab. Dr. Brink had written to me that the medical advice was quite unfavorable for continuing the research on isolation. I thought I knew the specific origin of the negative pressure, and which was influential. In addition, some in the company had never been sympathetic in the long search, because how could the company make a profit from treating a rare disease, even if the project were successful. My faith and that of Dr. Major in the potential worthwhileness to the company of a vitamin necessary for life probably kept us willful. I doubted that Dr. Major would stop my project in my absence, and he did not. On my return, he said something like, "Just take it easy!" After only a brief time, a few crystals of the vitamin were visible in a centrifuge tube, and could be witnessed by all including George Merck and other executives.

In retrospect, I believe that we would have succeeded to isolate vitamin B_{12} without the advent of *L. lactis* Dorner, because we were so conscious of the need of correlating some property with activity. This property became the red color, which was not far away. However, the microbial assay of Mary Shorb, which was ultimately expanded at Merck by Dr. Hendlin and Dr. Woodruff, was important.

To call the red crystalline substance the antipernicious anemia factor was unsatisfactory. The expression was too long and cumbersome and I sought a new name. Although a number of names were considered, I preferred the name vitamin B with the next unused number in vitamin nomenclature as the subscript. A new search of the literature and a check with Dr. Crane of Chemical Abstracts revealed no publication or unpublished abstract recording the name, vitamin B_{12}. Neither Dr. Crane nor I could have known that Professor Hauge of Purdue University had a manuscript in press with the expression vitamin B_{12}. The announcement of "Crystalline Vitamin B_{12}" by Ed Rickes, Norman Brink, Frank Koniuszy, Tom Wood and myself appeared in the issue of April 16, 1948 of *Science*. Professor Hauge told me some months later that when he saw our paper in *Science,* he changed all the 2's to 3's in the galley of his paper and which subsequently appeared with the expression "vitamin B_{13}."

As time passed after the first clinical tests on vitamin B_{12}, information concerning the discovery had apparently started to "leak" out of Columbia. In a fortuitous meeting of each other on the boardwalk of Atlantic City during a scientific meeting, Dr. Fritz Lipmann asked me if we had indeed discovered a new vitamin. The handling of the new medical information was different in policy at Columbia than at Merck. Publication had become timely, and not to do so was like trying to hide a building on fire.

There might have been just one joint paper in *Science* on vitamin B_{12} for the combined chemical, microbiological and clinical data. Instead, I prepared drafts for three companion manuscripts to be submitted for publication side by side in the same issue of *Science*. One manuscript was for ourselves at Merck, one was for Mary Shorb, and one was for Randolph West. The three manuscripts were completed by the appropriate parties and submitted together.

As we at Merck prepared the final draft of the chemical paper, we realized the significance of revealing that the crystalline vitamin B_{12} was red in color. As soon as this fact was known, any other group elsewhere with an advanced or stalemated isolation could within days or weeks complete the isolation, simply by watching for the development of the red band and then by following the band down columns for separation by color alone. Clinical assays were hardly needed at all except for confirmation of activities, and the microbiological assay need not be available. Also, we had observed that when fractions containing vitamin B_{12} reached a given but low level of purity, the substance crystallized out of an aqueous solvent mixture with the greatest of ease. Such a high crystallizing characteristic combined with the knowledge of the red color greatly benefited other laboratories to renew isolation or complete final isolations. I recall that Merck executives provided, for business reasons, prepublication knowledge of our success on the isolation of the red crystalline vitamin B_{12} and its extraordinary clinical activity in the successful treatment of pernicious anemia. Such prepublication data gave another time-advantage to others. . . .

Since most of us on this project were originally trained in organic chemistry, the isolation of the red vitamin was not the end of the project, but only the beginning of the chemistry. We made pioneering contributions to the structure of vitamin B_{12} as documented by 28 publications during 1948-1956. We elucidated with scientific priorities the benzimidazole and its riboside as well as the phosphate of the riboside. We also correctly identified the Dg-1-amino-2-propanol and synthesized this fragment in the correct optically active form. . . .

In summary, the discovery of the red crystalline vitamin B_{12} can be said to have occurred in an intellectual environment of mixed opinions and under experimental conditions which were at best precarious on many crucial occasions. . . . If vitamin B_{12} were unknown today, it is likely that the current management of research including proposals to be accepted or rejected, budget actions, market analyses, panels, diversified committees, hospital committees, safety regulations, and governmental procedures would constitute very different scenes in which the antipernicious anemia factor would have to be pursued to eventual discovery of the red crystalline vitamin.

Simultaneously, independent studies were being carried out without benefit of a microbiological assay at the Glaxo Laboratories in England by E. Lester Smith, who was also attempting to isolate the *antipernicious anemia principle* from liver extracts by the then newly developed technique of partition chromatography. The biological activities of the substances isolated by Smith were tested in untreated pernicious anemia patients by C. C. Ungley. In a recent personal communication to the author, Lester Smith (Fig. 36) provided some of his recollections regarding the isolation of vitamin B_{12} at Glaxo:

Preliminary work towards isolation of "Anti-Pernicious Anaemia Factor" (APAF) was started in 1937 but had to be put aside during the war years for more urgent projects, including penicillin. So it was not resumed till 1946. Meanwhile, Synge had invented a powerful new tool, partition chromatography, applied initially to separation of acylated aminoacids. I was immediately impressed with its potential for the APAF problem, and did find time then to try out the technique, and showed that it worked well with the lower fatty acids. It would need modification for my main problem, but I reckoned then that butanol as solvent might work for liver extracts,

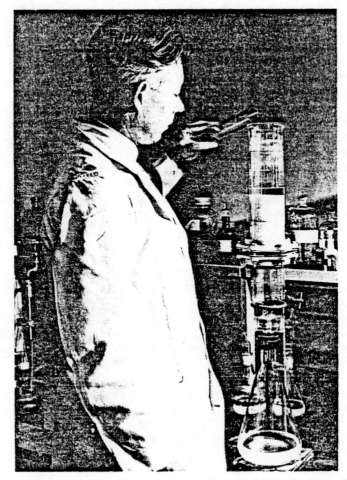

Figure 36.   E. Lester Smith in his laboratory at Glaxo in the 1940's. (Reproduced with permission of Glaxo Laboratories, Ltd., Greenford, Middlesex, England.)

and so it proved. At the earliest attempts a pink band showed up on the columns, along with brown and yellow ones. I recall Prof. A. R. Todd (now Lord Todd) visiting the Glaxo Research Laboratories at that time and being shown one of these columns. He dampened our excitement over the pink band, prophesying that this would turn out to be an adventitious pigment, and that the active factor, probably colorless, would be hidden in one of the other bands.

In any event a column with several distinct coloured zones was an embarrassment for testing. At that time we relied exclusively on clinical assays with human pernicious anaemia patients in relapse, carried out for us by Dr. C. Ungley at Newcastle-on Tyne. How long would it take to find enough subjects for reliable tests on, say, six fractions? As it happened, the answer was many anxious months, for just at that time the supply of untreated patients started to dry up. Also an early misleading test caused me to overestimate consistently the potency of my fractions, so that most of them had to be tested again at higher doses. To compound the exasperation, my research samples had of necessity to be accorded lower priority than clinical tests of the potency of commercial batches of our liver extract. Eventually of course, the tests did establish that activity lay in the pink fraction, and from then on, colour could be used to guide fractionation. For some time longer, however, we could not get beyond the stage of this amorphous pink powder; because it had a fairly constant potency from batch to batch, and resisted further concentration we supposed it must be nearly pure; in fact, as we later realised, it contained only around 1 percent of vitamin B_{12}. On account of heavy losses of initial potency during purification to this stage, we never had enough material to spare for really bold attempts at further purification, despite the many tons of liver that had been committed to this project.

I had in fact achieved about 10-fold further increase in potency when the bombshell dropped in the form of the historic note in *Science* from the Merck Laboratories, recording isolation of crystalline vitamin B_{12}. Another week of intensive work brought my material also to the crystalline state, and I was able to announce this a few days later and to show a slide of the crystals in a paper I was scheduled to read at the meeting of the Biochemical Society in Oxford. This was the only occasion I recall during some decades of attendance at the Society's meetings, when a paper was greeted by spontaneous applause. It later became clear that the Merck team had delayed publication for some months. Nevertheless, the scientific community graciously accepted the two independent publications as virtually simultaneous; this was partly because they represent the culmination of more than 20 years work by many research groups since Minot and Murphy first showed that liver extracts contained the APAF, and partly perhaps because my team lacked the microbiological assay that helped the Americans, and had to struggle along guided only by unreliable tests on human patients; that really seized the scientific imagination!

The history of vitamin B_{12} is littered with near-misses. Back in the late 1930's Laland and Klem in Norway already had an orange-pink active concentrate. With hindsight one can see how this might have been purified to the crystalline stage even without chromatography. Later, Short, working in Boots Research Laboratories in Nottingham, England, got a pink fraction but saw no hope of securing enough clinical tests to see if it was the active one. Petrow's team at British Drug Houses, and Wijmenga in Holland were close on our heels with isolation of vitamin B_{12}.

I remarked in an early paper that solutions of my concentrate had the colour of cobalt salts—but that certainly did not suggest to me that we were looking for an organic cobalt complex; no compounds even remotely resembling the cobalamins were known at the time. Later, however, I did get another indication, and this is a story I have not told previously. I decided to sacrifice a little of my precious material to see if it contained any ash, and I carried out the incineration in a porcelain crucible; the stuff disappeared without trace—or *almost* without trace, for I did see in one corner of the crucible a tiny blue flash that was gone before I could be sure I had really seen it. This time I did suspect a trace of cobalt fusing into the glaze of the crucible. But there was no weighable ash and I dismissed the phenomenon as probably due to impurity, instead of reasoning that the APAF itself contained cobalt, and that my preparation must still be very far from pure. Of course when we finally came to analyze the crystalline material, we quickly detected the presence of cobalt and phosphorus, and indeed were first to publish this, though we realised the Merck team must have been aware of the facts.

We were also first to record chromatographic separation of two forms of B_{12} (cyano- and hydroxycobalamin, as we later realised) though unfortunately we just missed spotting that the one could be converted into the other with cyanide, even though we had a clue that should have been followed up. But of course, what we all missed on our side of the Atlantic was an economic process for production of vitamin B_{12} by fermentation.

Isolation of vitamin B_{12} was only the beginning; it proved to be the most interesting vitamin ever. Its chemistry, and that of analogues, antagonists and coenzyme forms, its biochemistry, modes of absorption and physiological action, its nutritional and medical functions—all these gave rise to innumerable scientific papers over the next 20 years and more. As I remarked in an after-dinner speech at one of the long succession of vitamin B_{12} conferences: "This B_{12} isn't just a vitamin—it's a fraternity!"

Almost simultaneously in April of 1948, the American team at Merck headed by Folkers, and Lester Smith at Glaxo in England reported that the antipernicious anemia substance had been isolated from liver extracts. In an announcement as dramatic as Minot and Murphy's original report in 1926, Rickes et al. of the Merck Laboratories in the United States (Fig. 37) reported that they had isolated the *L. lactis* Dorner growth factor from liver extracts in the form of small red crystalline needles. They named the substance vitamin B_{12}.[345] In a recent personal communication to the author, Edward L. Rickes recalled the initial events surrounding the first isolation and crystallization of vitamin B_{12} by the Merck group in 1948:

At Merck & Co., Inc., I have been extremely fortunate to have had the opportunity of working on problems of great scientific interest and also of value to people. Our previous work on biotin, rhizopterin and pantothenic acid paved the way for the relatively quick isolation of B_{12}. Since that time there have been other problems but of course none of them have been as rewarding as the B_{12} crystallization.

I had just completed an alumina chromatograph with a fermentation extract being adsorbed. The effluent was quite red and gave a very high potency fraction when assayed on the L.L.D. (*Lactobacillus lactis* Dorner) assay. Tom Wood, very shortly thereafter, chromatographed an extract of liver powder with the same type alumina. The red effluent fraction was very noticeable and similar to my column. Tom and I, standing by the column, shook hands and said, "It sure looks as though we are finally on the right track." This occurred sometime in June or July; by December, the active compound was crystallized.

At a morning conference, it was decided not to send my 5.3 mg. L.L.D. concentrate sample to Dr. West, P&S (Columbia) for clinical testing. Left with this sample and having returned early from lunch, I decided to reprecipitate it. I dissolved the sample in water and added several drops of acetone. At this point, I was interrupted by a young microbiologist with whom we were doing some assay work. We talked for about 15-30 minutes. After he left, I went to the bench to resume my precipitation and stopped short. One of the most beautiful sights that a chemist is ever privileged to see, was the glint of several crystals sparkling in the light. I held the centrifuge tube to the light and watched the crystals form, after which I shakingly placed the tube in an Erlenmeyer and allowed the solution to stand. I went into Dick Boos' lab and told him what had happened. We both stood and admired the crystals glistening in the tube. A total of 3.2 mg. was recovered from the centrifuge tube on December 11, 1947.

A small amount of this was immediately submitted for analysis with much speculation on the metal ion content. Dick Boos soon gave us the answer. "Ed," he

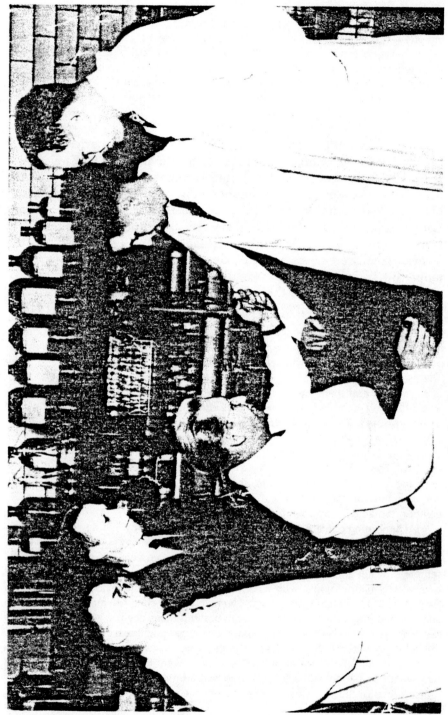

See legend on the opposite page.

said, "we have been neighbors and friends a long time but I never thought you would have a purple ash." Of course, the presence of cobalt was quickly confirmed.

At the same time as the initial publication of the Merck investigators,[345] Randolph West at Columbia University reported the therapeutic effects of the first administration of the newly isolated crystalline vitamin B_{12} to three patients with untreated pernicious anemia.[423] He found that the substance was exceedingly potent in small amounts and led to a hematological remission in these patients. Simultaneously, Shorb[371] reported that the newly crystallized vitamin B_{12} was the essential "growth factor" for *L. lactis* Dorner.

Only eight days after the publication of Rickes et al.'s discovery of crystalline vitamin B_{12},[345] Lester Smith at the Glaxo Laboratories in England published his report in which he purified two red "antipernicious anemia" pigments by chromatography from ox liver extracts.[375] These pigments were amorphous solids with the "color of cobalt salts," a molecular weight of less than 10,000, and were effective in the treatment of pernicious anemia.

In a subsequent paper several weeks after Smith's announcement of purification of two red "antipernicious anemia" pigments, Smith and Parker[376] reported that they had purified a "pink" compound by chromatography from ox liver. This pink compound was then crystallized from acetone and formed red needles similar to those found by the Merck group.[345] Smith[377] was also the first to report the presence of cobalt in crystalline vitamin B_{12} and noted that cobalt had not been previously detected in an isolated compound of natural origin. Reference was made to the earlier agricultural work of Martin[283] indicating that cobalt-containing substances might have an essential role in normal erythropoiesis.

Studies of poultry nutrition again entered the pernicious anemia story at this point and at first appeared to have little or no connection with human disease. During the war-time period when there was a scarcity of animal feed for poultry, it was observed that chickens fed on a vegetable diet alone grew poorly. This growth defect was ameliorated by the feeding of animal protein, and the term *animal protein factor* was given to this growth substance. It was subsequently shown that dried cow manure was an unusually potent source of the animal protein factor. Later it was found that during the summer months when chicks ingested food materials contaminated with their own feces, they had less need for the animal protein factor than otherwise.

These observations combined with the activity shown to be present in cow manure suggested that microorganisms contained in the

---

Figure 37. The team of scientists at Merck & Co. who in 1948 were the first to report the isolation and crystallization of vitamin B_{12} from liver extracts. Left to right are Frank R. Koniuszy, Karl A. Folkers, Edward L. Rickes, Norman G. Brink, and Thomas R. Wood. (From the Merck Report, October 1952, p. 3. Reproduced with permission of Merck & Co., Rahway, N.J.)

feces might be capable of synthesizing the animal protein factor. This microbial capability was reported in 1948 by Stokstad et al.[382] who found that a rod-shaped nonmotile organism in hen feces could synthesize an animal protein factor active in chicks and that concentrates of this microbially produced material were effective in producing hematological remissions in untreated pernicious anemia patients. Stokstad et al.[382] hypothesized that the bacterial extract contained forms or complexes of the antipernicious anemia factor.

With the knowledge that the animal protein factor found in hen feces and in cow manure were probably the same substance as the antipernicious anemia factor, it became apparent that microorganisms could synthesize substances that had potent hematological activity in untreated pernicious anemia patients. The next step in this sequence was taken by Rickes et al.[346] who demonstrated that from the fermentation liquors of *Streptomyces griseus*, a microorganism used for the commercial production of streptomycin, crystalline vitamin B_{12} could be isolated. This discovery facilitated the large-scale production of vitamin B_{12} from microbial sources, which is today the commercial process for manufacturing vitamin B_{12}.

Following the isolation of crystalline vitamin B_{12},[141,345,375] Lester Smith brought several crystals of the vitamin to Dorothy Crowfoot Hodgkin, a brilliant x-ray crystallographer at Oxford. In a series of elegant x-ray diffraction studies performed between 1950 and 1956 and involving more than 10 million calculations, Hodgkin et al.[210-212] elucidated the molecular structure of vitamin B_{12}. In doing so, Hodgkin et al. identified a hitherto undescribed biological entity that formed the heart of the vitamin B_{12} molecule, namely, the corrin nucleus. This discovery helped to make possible the many advances in corrinoid chemistry that have occurred subsequently.[332] In 1956, Hodgkin et al.[212] reported that the vitamin B_{12} molecule was spherical with all the chemically reactive groups on the surface. It was built around the two planes of the key imidazole nucleus that were nearly at right angles to each other. They postulated the formula of vitamin B_{12} to be $C_{63}H_{88}O_{14}N_{14}PCo$.

In a recent personal note to the author, Dorothy Hodgkin (Fig. 38) recalled some of the highlights of her pioneering experiments:

It was a Friday in April 1948 that Dr. Lester Smith brought the first crystals he had obtained of the antipernicious anaemia factor to Oxford. He was reporting on his work to a meeting of the Biochemical Society the following morning. He brought the crystals with a view to their examination by Dr. R. C. Spiller, in the Department of Mineralogy, since the Merck chemists had recorded in *Science* the refractive indices of the crystals they had obtained a few months earlier. It was desirable to check that Lester Smith's crystals had the same refractive indices. The crystals, as Lester Smith first showed them to me, were very small and imbedded in a little gluey material. I could see that they were red and also that they were pleochroic, and I asked to take x-ray photographs of them. The first one was taken overnight and developed the next morning; the second photograph was taken during the meeting.

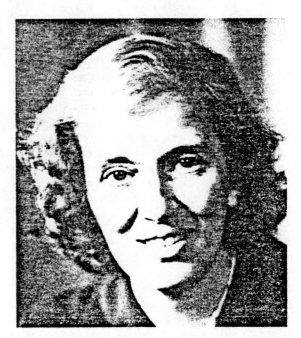

Figure 38. Dorothy C. Hodgkin (1910-   ). (Reproduced with permission of the Nobel Foundation, Stockholm, Sweden.)

Before Dr. Lester Smith left Oxford it was possible to tell him that the crystals were almost certainly orthorhombic and that, from the dimensions of the unit cell, the molecular weight must be no more than half the figure he had quoted as likely in the talk he gave, of the order of 1500, rather than 3000. I remember very well Bill Pirie, who believes in a critical attitude to all scientific observations, joking at the meeting with Lester Smith, "Perhaps the active substance was just some small impurity on the surface of the crystals." But the activity, of course, was already much higher than that of most pharmaceutical materials. I said I felt sure that the striking pleochroism meant that there was something like a porphyrin nucleus in the crystals, and this inclined me to think they were the really active material. I did not immediately think of working on the structure of the antipernicious anemia factor; at that moment I had no chemical information about it at all. Lester Smith improved the crystallisation, and the Merck chemists sent over some of their material so that I could compare the characteristics of x-ray photographs taken from both preparations. They were clearly essentially the same.

It was, I think, in May that I had a telephone call during the lunch hour at home from Dr. MacRae of Glaxo Laboratories. I had with me at lunch a visitor from Denmark, Dr. Bodil Jerslev, who had just arrived to work in Oxford for some months. Dr. MacRae said, "We have found cobalt in the crystals of the antipernicious anemia factor. The amount corresponds to one atom for your molecular weight. There's a heavy atom for you—could you not work on the structure?" It was very exciting news indeed and did encourage me to work on the structure, though I was a little hesitant since cobalt seemed to me rather a small heavy atom in relation to the size of the molecule as a whole. Dr. MacRae had raised the idea, because the Glaxo chemists had been our colleagues earlier in the study of the structure of penicillin, and they knew our requirements: good crystals which would give many diffraction effects and, preferably, crystals containing replaceable heavy atoms, from which we could form an isomorphous series. By the calculation of three-dimensional Patterson maps we hoped to find the positions of the heavy atoms, and it was easy to find them in the penicillin case, because we could replace potassium by rubidium in the salts we had.

So the next very exciting moment I remember in the B_{12} story was the calculation of the first three-dimensional Patterson series from the crystals of the antipernicious anemia factor itself, alone. The intensities were measured by Dr. June Broomhead (later Lindsay), a post-doctoral fellow, and the calculations were carried out by Miss Gittus in Liverpool. She had been Comrie's assistant on the penicillin calculations and had access to punched card machines. I think she did it for something like £100. The maps showed immediately three very heavy peaks, which defined the relative positions of the cobalt atoms in the crystals, and around each peak we could see in the Patterson map an octahedron of smaller peaks, which clearly defined the relative positions of atoms attached to the cobalt atom. We could see still more than this. It seemed to us clear that the structure was soluble by x-ray methods involving only data from the one crystal form. However, we were in for trouble later! The relative positions of the cobalt atoms provided a rather imperfect definition of the phase relations and the first electron density maps we saw proved very complicated to interpret. Our computing methods also were very primitive.

Very slowly, and partly with the help of studies of other near isomorphous crystals containing selenium attached to cobalt, we began to recognize that the group surrounding the cobalt atom was not exactly a regular porphyrin. It would be impossible here to give any account of the complicated stages through which we and others passed. Work on the B_{12} structure proceeded in a number of chemical laboratories and groups attached to the cobalt atom, the benzimidazole, sugar, phosphate and cyanide groups were identified. The Merck chemists encouraged Dr. John White to carry out x-ray analytical calculations on their crystals. As we both became confused about our results, we went into collaboration rather than competition and compared all our conclusions. With hindsight now, we could have solved the structure on data from cyanocobalamin crystals alone.

We were, in fact, very greatly assisted by the isolation in 1953 of a degradation product, the hexacarboxylic acid, by Jack Cannon, working with Todd and Johnson in Cambridge. The crystals of the hexacarboxylic acid formed during Jack Cannon's summer holiday from a solution containing a mixture of solvents. We borrowed the whole preparation from Cambridge in our search for a few suitable crystals, before returning it to them for further chemical studies. I remember a letter from Alan Johnson, warning me that we should not spend too much time on the crystals, since they were very impure and my replying, half joking, "Your whole preparation may be impure, but our one crystal is giving very beautiful diffraction effects, and we have nearly completed the measurements." This one crystal was studied by Jenny Pickworth (Glusker), a D. Phil. student, and Dr. John Robertson, and proved much simpler to interpret than the B_{12} crystals themselves. From the first Patterson it was easy to define the cobalt positions and the electron density map following showed the same odd structure of the nucleus we had dimly seen in the other maps. From then on, the structure analysis progressed very rapidly, much more rapidly than we could have dreamed. The following year it was possible to write the whole vitamin structure.

The first certain evidence of the structure of the nucleus was obtained in May 1954. I had been asked the preceding autumn to give the Congress Lecture at the Third Meeting of the International Union of Crystallography in Paris about the work on vitamin B_{12}. I had refused, since I did not think we knew enough about the structure for such a serious occasion. However, in May, the organizers asked me again, at just the moment when we knew our ideas about the structure of the nucleus were correct, and we accepted with delight. At about the same time, Dr. Ken True-blood passed through the laboratory, and offered to do calculations for us on SWAC, an early electronic computer in California, absolutely free. We tested him out on calciferol first (same space group) and then sent him a structure factor calculation, which included placing all of the atoms in the nucleus of the hexacarboxylic acid, in August, while we went off to Paris to enjoy our Congress. We returned from Paris to find a great mass of figures waiting for us—the next refinement stage of the electron density map. There was a meeting of the British Association in Oxford at the time, at which we had set up some models showing all we thought we knew about the B_{12} structure. It always makes me feel a little odd to think that the pile of computer output that we put on the same table included evidence of all the rest of the structure, as we realised when we worked carefully through it in the following months.

Perhaps the next most exciting events occurred with the analysis of the B_{12} co-enzyme by Dr. Galen Lenhert. By then we were experienced and Galen Lenhert was a very beautiful worker, so the course of the analysis was more straightforward. It was not so difficult to understand the first electron density maps phased on the cobalt positions only and, at the second round, we began to perceive the nature of the new group attached to the cobalt in place of the cyanide of our first crystals. It took a day to realise what it was. Curiously, I looked through the maps with Galen in the morning, and we drew the structure out without fully realising the force of the pattern we drew. I realised it walking along Piccadilly with Donald Woods on the way to a Royal Society party that evening, and he was the first person whom I told the astonishing fact that the cobalt was attached to the carbon atom of deoxyadenosine.

For her contributions, Dorothy Hodgkin was awarded the Nobel Prize in Chemistry in 1964. Not only was she a pioneer in her work involving the molecular structure of vitamin B_{12}, but her use of x-ray crystallographic methods to determine the structure of a pure biological substance paved the way for the subsequent use of x-ray crystallography by Perutz and Kendrew that ultimately led to the discovery of the molecular structure of hemoglobin and myoglobin.

Radioactive vitamin B_{12} was synthesized by Chaiet et al.[87] in 1950 and by Rosenblum and Woodbury[351] in 1951, who added radioactive cobalt to fermentations of *S. griseus*. Their investigations made possible many subsequent experiments utilizing the isotopic form of the vitamin. Another major advance in the story of vitamin B_{12} and pernicious anemia was made by Barker et al.[27] who in 1958 isolated the biologically active form of vitamin B_{12}. This was called 5'-deoxyadenosylcobalamin, or coenzyme B_{12}. It is the form in which vitamin B_{12} is believed to be stored within the body, primarily in the liver,[403] and it functions as a prosthetic group for the enzyme methylmalonyl-CoA mutase.[170,373]

The most recent aspect of the vitamin B_{12} and pernicious anemia saga occurred in 1972, 46 years after the original observations of Minot and Murphy. Robert B. Woodward (Fig. 39) of the Department of Chemistry at Harvard University, already a Nobel Laureate in Chemistry in 1965 as a result of his earlier contributions to organic chemistry and the synthesis of naturally occurring substances, achieved the total synthesis of vitamin B_{12}.[442] In collaboration with Eschenmoser in Zurich, Woodward set as his goal the synthesis of

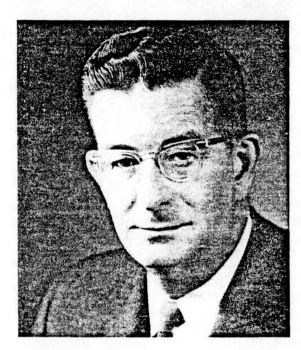

Figure 39. Robert B. Woodward (1917-   ). (Reproduced with permission of the Nobel Foundation, Stockholm, Sweden.)

cobyric acid, a compound identical to the nuclear portion of vitamin B_{12}. Starting with carbon, nitrogen, and oxygen, and including a unique process of cobaltization, Woodward synthesized cobyric acid. With the addition of the appropriate side chains, the molecule of vitamin B_{12} itself was completely synthesized.

Recently Robert B. Woodward communicated to the author some of the challenges in organic chemistry that were encountered in the efforts to synthesize vitamin B_{12}:

In accepting that challenge, my colleagues and I—as well as Professor Eschenmoser and his group in Zürich—were taken up in an absorbing adventure which in a sense almost became a way of life; Professor Eschenmoser put it well when he asserted jokingly to an interviewer: "He (speaking of me) is sorry that it's finished!" I believe it is fair to say that the investigation was unique in more than one way. It engaged one hundred collaborators from nineteen countries, presented an example of splendidly pleasurable and fruitful international collaboration, and was pursued intensively over a period of eleven years. The chemical intricacies encountered, and the experimental skill and intellectual élan mobilized (the latter by no means alone by Professor Eschenmoser and myself), were certainly larger in measure and quality than any we had been presented with in our earlier work.

Synthetic investigation is the core of contemporary organic chemistry. It is the arena in which principles and methods are put to the most rigorous test, refined, sharpened and defined in scope. But even more important is the opportunity which such work presents for extension and innovation, both in theory and in practice. The work which culminated in the synthesis of vitamin B_{12} provided what is almost certainly the most spectacular known example of these truths. For the discovery of the principle of orbital symmetry conservation, with its dramatic consequences for all chemistry, arose directly from the B_{12} investigation.

MILESTONES IN PERNICIOUS ANEMIA

Year	Person	Contribution
1824	Combe	First description of what appears to be pernicious anemia, and first mention that it may be related to a disorder of the digestive system.
1849	Addison	First detailed description of patient with severe, probably pernicious anemia.
1851	Möller	First description of glossitis in *Diphyllobothrium latum*-induced anemia.
1855	Addison	Additional account of severe *idiopathic* anemia.
1860	Flint	First suggestion that pernicious anemia may be due to a disorder of the *gastric tubuli*.
1870	Fenwick	First accurate and illustrated description of atrophic gastritis and physiological documentation of achlorhydria. Fenwick's patient may have also had pernicious anemia.
1872	Biermer	Description of a probably heterogeneous group of anemic individuals, and the first mention of the term *progressive pernicious anemia* as a clinical entity exemplified by these anemic patients.
1875	Pepper	First description of the bone marrow in pernicious anemia.
1876-77	Quincke	First description of poikilocytes in pernicious anemia blood.
1877	Cohnheim	First recognition that the hyperplasia of the bone marrow in pernicious anemia was due to increased numbers of erythroid precursors.
1877	Hayem	First description of the giant macrocyte in pernicious anemia.
1878	Eichhorst	First description of the microcyte in pernicious anemia blood.
1880	Ehrlich	First designation of the abnormal erythroid precursor in pernicious anemia as the megaloblast.
1883	Laache	Early monograph on pernicious anemia, and first illustration of the macrocyte in the blood.
1884	Leichtenstern	Initial account of neurological abnormalities in pernicious anemia.

1886	Cahn and von Mering	First description of actual gastric analysis in patients with severe anemia, and observation that achlorhydria was often associated with severe anemia.
1887	Lichtheim	First full description of neurological abnormalities, including sensory changes, in pernicious anemia.
1903	Cabot	Description of ring bodies in erythrocytes in pernicious anemia.
1905	Ehrlich and Lazarus	Detailed description of the megaloblast and observations of its unique staining properties.
1921	Levine and Ladd	One of the first accurate studies documenting achlorhydria as a *sine qua non* for the confident diagnosis of pernicious anemia. Also an early genetic study.
1923	Hurst	Further observations regarding possible etiological relationships between achlorhydria and pernicious anemia.
1925	Whipple and Robscheit-Robbins	Observations that liver was a potent hematopoietic substance in probably iron-deficient dogs.
1926	Murphy	First documented hospital case of a patient with severe pernicious anemia treated successfully with liver.
1926	Minot and Murphy	First published reports of the efficacy of liver therapy in pernicious anemia.
1927	Peabody	First report of the conversion of megaloblastic to normoblastic erythropoiesis in the marrow of pernicious anemia patients treated with liver.
1928	Cohn et al.	Production of a biologically potent aqueous extract of liver.
1928-29	Castle et al.	Initial accounts of gastric intrinsic factor and its relationship to the etiology and pathogenesis of pernicious anemia.
1948	Rickes et al. and Smith	Isolation and crystallization of vitamin B_{12}, the *antipernicious anemia principle*, from liver extracts.
1950-56	Hodgkin et al.	Determination of the crystalline structure of vitamin B_{12} molecule by x-ray diffraction.
1958	Barker et al.	Discovery of coenzyme B_{12} (5′-deoxyadenosylcobalamin).
1972	Woodward and Eschenmoser	Total synthesis of vitamin B_{12}.

CHAPTER 2

CLINICAL AND HEMATOLOGICAL FEATURES OF PERNICIOUS ANEMIA

Although it is said to occur more commonly in Scandinavian and "English-speaking" people,[273] pernicious anemia has been described in all racial groups[88,387] and is believed to occur more frequently in males than in females.[88,387] The incidence of pernicious anemia in the general population is approximately 2 to 6 per 1000.[88,387]

To date, the classical description of a patient with severe untreated pernicious anemia given by Addison in 1849[8] and 1855[9] remains one of the most vivid and accurate accounts. Although some patients present in the florid manner described by Addison, in many other patients the onset is insidious, and they may complain initially of mild weakness, fatigue, lethargy, and pallor similar to that found in many other kinds of anemia. Occasionally shortness of breath and edema are observed and may be related to congestive heart failure as a result of the anemia. In certain patients, the lack of symptoms in relation to the degree of severity of the anemia can be impressive. Occasionally the diagnosis of pernicious anemia may either be overlooked or in some instances discovered accidentally in the course of an evaluation of some other disorder or complaint. Distaste for meat, bloating, and dyspeptic symptoms are commonly observed. Premature graying or whitening of the hair,[189] low-set ears, acromegaloid facies,[123] and blue eyes have been noted as prominent anthropomorphic features in patients with pernicious anemia, but they are inconstant findings. A lemon yellow color of the skin has been said to be characteristic, although waxy pallor is seen more frequently in severe cases. In some instances, frank icterus may occur and is due to hyper-

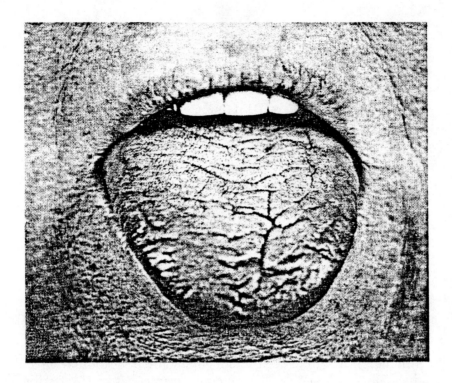

Plate 1. *Top.* Beefy-red tongue devoid of papillations in a patient with pernicious anemia. (Photograph courtesy of Dr. Muriel C. Meyers.) *Bottom.* Smooth, pale white, clean-appearing tongue in a patient with pernicious anemia. (Photograph courtesy of Dr. Muriel C. Meyers.)

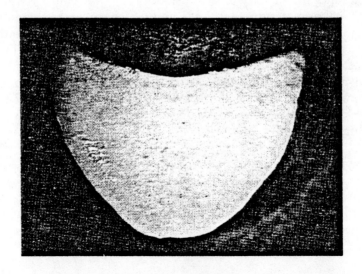

bilirubinemia resulting in large part from intramedullary destruction of erythrocytes and erythroid precursors.[277] Vitiligo may also be found.

Glossitis is particularly common in pernicious anemia and has been known since the time of Möller[301] and Barclay[26] in the 1850s. A painful beefy red tongue devoid of papillae has been described as typical of pernicious anemia (Plate 1). Actually, this type of tongue may be seen less frequently than a pale, smooth, clean-appearing tongue with loss of papillae on the surface and sides (Plate 1). Hepatomegaly is occasionally found, and on rare occasions the spleen tip can be palpated. Pitting edema of the extremities is seen in severe cases and may be associated with congestive heart failure.

Neurological symptoms of subacute combined degeneration of the spinal cord may be the presenting manifestations of vitamin B_{12} deficiency in some patients, and numbness and tingling in the extremities may be particularly distressing for certain individuals. Loss of vibratory and position sense in the lower extremities is a frequent physical finding. Mental aberrations in the form of psychotic manifestations, so-called megaloblastic madness,[374] are seen in some individuals. In others, mild aberrations of otherwise normal behavior for the particular individual may be seen. On rare occasions a patient may demonstrate the neurological complications of pernicious anemia with very low levels of vitamin B_{12} in the spinal fluid and peripheral blood but have little or no anemia. In some instances, a careful dietary history may reveal that such a patient has ingested either folic acid or foods rich in folate.

Visual disturbances may occur,[93,106,235] and optic atrophy,[93,106,235] retinal hemorrhages,[45,282] and Roth spots may be observed on funduscopic examination. Anosmia may also be found in pernicious anemia, and the patient may be unable to taste or smell food properly. Azospermia resulting in infertility has been noted, as has amenorrhea.

In typical cases laboratory studies, in addition to hematological abnormalities, reveal serum vitamin B_{12} levels (*Euglena gracilis* or *Lactobacillus leichmannii*) generally less than 100 picograms/milliliter (normal 315 + 125 picograms/milliliter) and normal or elevated serum folate levels. The degree of severity of megaloblastosis in the marrow is usually, but not always, directly proportional to the degree of lowering of the serum B_{12} level. The serum iron and bilirubin are generally elevated and usually fall after treatment. Serum LDH levels are frequently elevated[199] and probably reflect intramedullary destruction of erythrocytes and megaloblasts that are known to have a high content of LDH in pernicious anemia.[385]

In some instances, the diagnosis of pernicious anemia may be unsuspected on the basis of peripheral blood examination alone, since the pancytopenia that occurs so frequently in severe cases can also occur in a variety of other hematological disorders including aplastic anemia, myelophthisic anemia, hypersplenism, subleukemic leukemia, and myelofibrosis with myeloid metaplasia. In severe cases where proerythroblasts and myelocytes are found in the peripheral blood, pernicious anemia can sometimes be misdiagnosed as eryth-roleukemia until the correct diagnosis is made after examination of the bone marrow and determination of serum vitamin B_{12} levels and gastric analysis. Occasionally, other types of nonnutritional macrocytic anemias with megaloblastoid-type erythropoiesis such as chronic erythremic myelosis have also been misdiagnosed as pernicious anemia[244] until the proper diagnostic studies have been obtained.

Determination of gastric acidity before and after maximal histamine stimulation[69,88] reveals (1) a substantially decreased volume of gastric juice having a thick, tenacious appearance; (2) absent acid secretion with failure of the pH to fall below 3.5 (achlorhydria); in

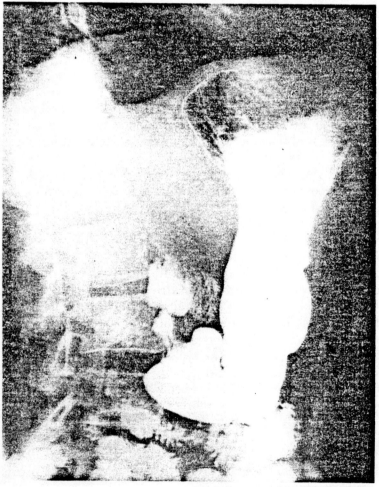

Figure 40. Radiographic demonstration of atrophic gastritis in a patient with pernicious anemia. Loss of gastric rugae is noted particularly in the fundus.

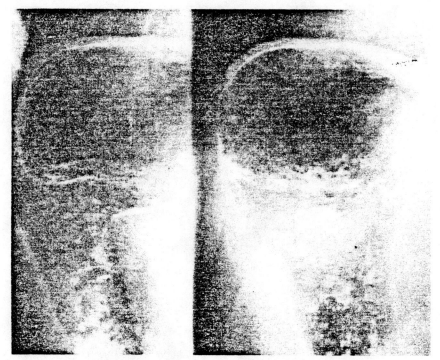

Figure 41. Gastric atrophy in pernicious anemia, showing loss of rugal folds in the fundus of the stomach.

many patients with pernicious anemia, the pH of the gastric juice remains at 6.0 or above after maximal histamine stimulation; (3) amounts of pepsin and rennin in the gastric juice are decreased; and (4) the intrinsic factor is markedly decreased or absent. To minimize the incidence of side effects of histamine, such as flushing, sweating, and a sense of warmth, betazole hydrochloride (Histalog, Lilly) can be used instead of histamine when performing a gastric acid stimulation test. The maximal histamine test should not be used in individuals who have an allergic history or coronary artery disease. Despite the gastric achlorhydria, serum gastrin levels are markedly increased in pernicious anemia,[188] indicating that the gastrin secreting cells of the stomach are not affected by the atrophic process and apparently remain susceptible to the regulatory control of acid and secretin.

Radiographic examination of the stomach may reveal atrophic gastritis as seen in Figures 40 and 41. Loss of rugal folds is especially prominent in the gastric fundus (Fig. 41). Gastric biopsies often reveal loss of parietal cells, loss of gastric rugae, and large epithelial cells with wrinkled nuclear membranes and prominent nucleoli (Fig. 42A). Variation in size and shape of gastric epithelial cells is seen. Gastric exfoliative cytology (Figs. 42B and 42C) may demonstrate large atypical epithelial cells described initially by Massey and Rubin[284] as "PA" cells.

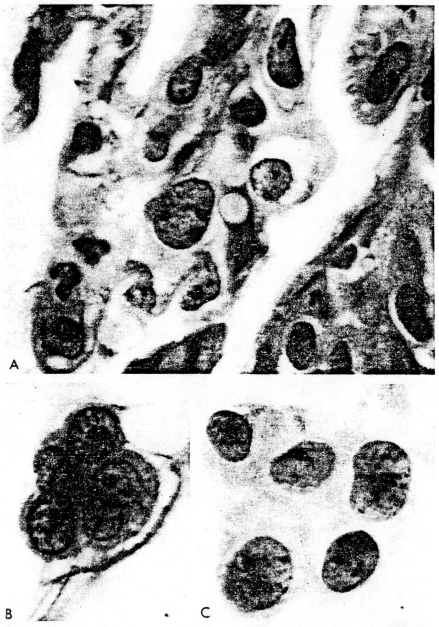

Figure 42. **A.** Gastric biopsy from a patient with pernicious anemia, stained with hematoxylin and eosin. Large atypical gastric columnar cells with prominent nucleoli and wrinkled nuclear membranes are seen. **B.** Large multinucleate gastric mucosal cell obtained by gastric exfoliative cytology from a patient with pernicious anemia. Prominent nucleoli are seen. (Papanicolaou stain.) **C.** Group of large atypical gastric epithelial cells from gastric washings in a patient with pernicious anemia. Prominent nucleoli and enlarged nuclei are seen. (Papanicolaou stain.)

Other disorders believed to have a basis in autoimmunity are sometimes seen in association with pernicious anemia. These include idiopathic myxedema, Hashimoto's thyroiditis, systemic lupus erythematosus, and rarely hypoadrenalism.[203] The author has also observed several pernicious anemia patients who have had a simultaneous warm-antibody Coombs-positive hemolytic anemia.

The relationship between pernicious anemia and acute leukemia is unclear, and it is uncertain whether a relationship does in fact exist. Between 1900 and 1910, cases of an ill-defined entity called *leukanemia* were reported by Von Leube, Parkes-Weber, Treadgold, and others.[244] Although these cases of *leukanemia* were originally thought to represent a transition from pernicious anemia to leukemia and in some instances a combination of pernicious anemia and acute leukemia, it is more likely that many of them represented examples of erythroleukemia.[244] The occurrence of acute leukemia in patients who have had pernicious anemia is believed to be very rare. In one patient reported by Zarafonetis et al.,[446] an unusual sequence of hematological disorders was observed, beginning with pernicious anemia, followed by polycythemia vera, and terminating in acute myeloblastic leukemia.

The following four cases illustrate typical clinical and morphological abnormalities as the anemia becomes progressively severe.

Case I   Minimal Pernicious Anemia

A 69-year-old man was in good health until two months prior to admission when he developed persistent right upper quadrant pain. On physical examination at the University of Michigan Medical Center, his blood pressure was 140/90 mm Hg, and pulse 100 per minute. Pertinent physical findings included splinting of the right upper quadrant, and palmar erythema. Laboratory test results included a hemoglobin of 14.4 gm%, hematocrit 42.4%, red blood cell count 3.82 million/mm³, mean corpuscular volume 111 cubic microns, mean corpuscular hemoglobin concentration 33.9%, reticulocyte count 2.0%, white blood cell count 11,100/mm³ with 92% polymorphonuclear leukocytes, 3% lymphocytes, and 5% monocytes. The serum folate was 30.5 ng/ml, serum B_{12} 50 pg/ml, and serum iron 89 μg/ml. A Schilling test demonstrated 0.57% excretion of radioactivity, and after the administration of intrinsic factor the excretion was 16%. An upper GI series showed a deformed gastric antrum. On gastroscopy, no evidence of atrophic gastritis was found, but the pylorus was severely deformed. The pH of gastric secretions was 6.0 both before and after histamine stimulation. A gastric biopsy revealed atrophic gastritis.

The peripheral blood of patients with pernicious anemia in the minimally anemic or even pre-anemic phase may disclose few abnormalities. Often, however, a generalized macrocytosis may be found (Fig. 43). In these cases the mean corpuscular volume of erythrocytes is generally greater than 100 cubic microns. Macroovalocytes are usually observed. Occasionally, hypersegmented macropolymorphonu-

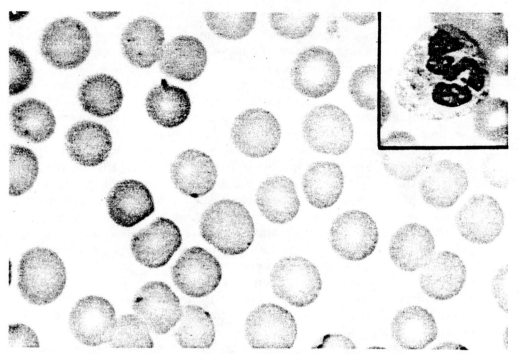

Figure 43. Peripheral blood from patient with minimal pernicious anemia. Generalized macrocytosis of erythrocytes is observed. Inset illustrates a hypersegmented macropolymorphonuclear leukocyte.

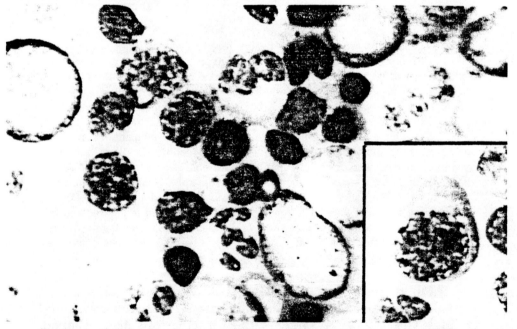

Figure 44. Bone marrow from patient with minimal pernicious anemia, showing focal attenuation of chromatin strands in intermediate normoblasts. Inset illustrates a large early intermediate macronormoblast with focal attenuation of chromatin strands and nucleocytoplasmic asynchrony.

clear leukocytes may be found (Fig. 43, inset). Multiple connections between adjacent nuclear lobes may be observed. Abnormalities in other peripheral blood leukocytes are usually not seen, and platelets appear normal on the peripheral film. Occasionally basophilic stippling of erythrocytes may be found.

The bone marrow at this stage when the serum vitamin B_{12} is low but the patient is only minimally anemic is said by some to be entirely normal. However, as exemplified by Case I, subtle abnormalities in both erythroid and granulocytic precursors can often be found. Proerythroblasts may be slightly increased in number, but overall the total number of erythroid precursors is within normal limits. Although frank megaloblasts are usually not present, the nuclear chromatin of many of the erythroid precursors frequently shows focal areas of attenuation of chromatin strands, as seen in Figure 44. In other erythroid precursors, evidence of nucleocytoplasmic asynchrony can be found (Fig. 44, inset) and at times unusually large macronormoblasts can be seen. The nuclear chromatin pattern in the erythroid precursors sometimes exhibits a "clockface" appearance.[238] Aberrant-appearing late macronormoblasts and late megaloblasts, as seen in more well developed cases of pernicious anemia, are usually not found at this stage.

Macropolymorphonuclear leukocytes with hypersegmented nuclei are sometimes seen in the bone marrow. In addition, as seen in

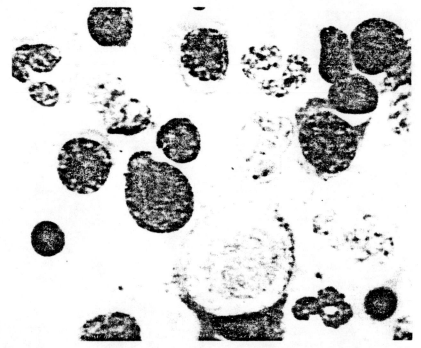

Figure 45. Bone marrow, minimal pernicious anemia, illustrating macronormoblastic erythropoiesis and giant bands with twisted and atypical nuclei, some of which have bulbous ends.

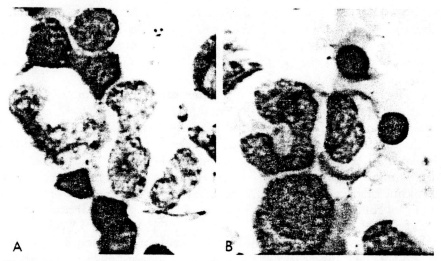

A   B

Figure 46. **A.** Giant metamyelocytes with bulbous ends of nuclei in a patient with minimal pernicious anemia. **B.** Giant atypical metamyelocyte with squared nuclear configuration and bulbous nuclear ends.

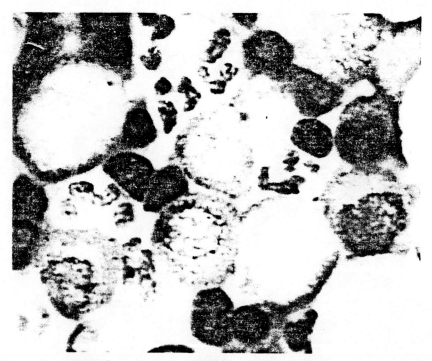

Figure 47. Increased numbers of eosinophil myelocytes in the bone marrow of a patient with minimal pernicious anemia.

Figure 45, giant "band" forms with unusual nuclear twistings can also be found. Some of the metamyelocytes are large and exhibit bulbous ends of their nuclei (Fig. 46). Increased numbers of eosinophil myelocytes may be found (Fig. 47). Abnormalities in megakaryocytes and plasma cells are usually not observed in these minimally anemic patients.

Case II   Mild Pernicious Anemia

A 28-year-old white woman was found to have a hematocrit of 35% two years prior to admission. The hematocrit steadily fell over the ensuing two years, but she felt well. After childbirth one year prior to admission, the hematocrit fell to 23%. She was treated with iron, and the hematocrit increased to 40%. Prior to admission she came to the emergency ward complaining of fever and cough. In addition to acute bronchitis she was found to have a hematocrit of 31% and an erythrocyte mean corpuscular volume of 112 cubic microns. The patient had an adequate dietary history, and the review of systems aside from premature hair loss was negative. On physical examination at the University of Michigan Medical Center her blood pressure was 90/70 mm Hg, the pulse 100 and regular. Pertinent physical findings included premature alopecia and slightly decreased papillations of the surface of the tongue. Laboratory test results included a hemoglobin of 11.5 gm%, hematocrit 34%, red blood cell count 3.0 million/mm^3, mean corpuscular volume 113.5 cubic microns, mean corpuscular hemoglobin concentration 33.8%, and a reticulocyte count of less than 1%. The white blood cell count was 3250/mm^3 with 52% polymorphonuclear leukocytes, 35% lymphocytes, 4% monocytes, 1% eosinophils, and 8% broken cells. Platelets were reduced in number on the peripheral film. The serum iron was 75 μg%, total iron binding capacity 306 μg%, serum B$_{12}$ 87 pg/ml, and serum folate 5.95 ng/ml. The Schilling test without intrinsic factor showed 0.52% excretion, and 18% excretion of radioactivity after the administration of intrinsic factor. The findings of an upper GI series were normal.

The peripheral blood of patients with mild pernicious anemia who have hemoglobin levels of approximately 11.0 grams show numerous large macroovalocytes and macrocytes (Fig. 48). The erythrocyte mean corpuscular volume is usually greater than 100 cubic microns. In addition to macroovalocytes, small microcytes may also be observed, and basophilic stippling of erythrocytes can be seen. Hypersegmented macropolymorphonuclear leukocytes with multiple connections between nuclear lobes are also observed (Fig. 48, inset). The platelets may appear reduced in number on inspection of the peripheral blood film. Abnormalities are usually not found in other peripheral blood cells. The white blood cell count and platelet count are usually normal or at the lower limits of normal at this stage of the anemia.

The bone marrow of patients with anemia at this stage shows clear evidence of developing megaloblastic changes in some of the erythroid precursors. Proerythroblasts may be slightly increased in

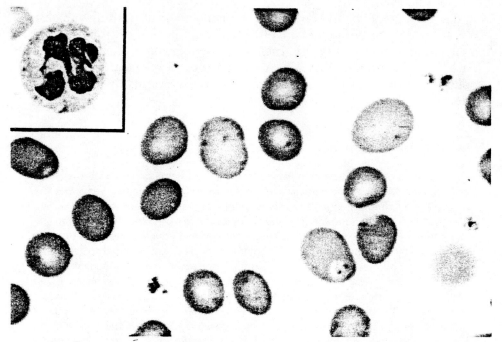

Figure 48. Peripheral blood from a patient with mild pernicious anemia, showing variation of size and shape of erythrocytes and macroovalocytes. *Inset:* macropolymorphonuclear leukocyte with nuclear hypersegmentation and multiple connections between nuclear lobes.

number. The majority of the erythroid precursors are early and late intermediate macronormoblasts (Fig. 49), and in many of them attenuation of chromatin strands and loss of chromatin aggregates that are characteristic of megaloblastic maturation can be observed (Fig. 49). There are usually normal numbers of erythroid precursors at this stage. Unusually large and binucleate erythroid precursors with megaloblastic chromatin pattern are seen infrequently (Fig. 49, inset). Some of the late macronormoblasts show aberrant-appearing "cloverleaf" nuclear chromatin patterns.

In cases where there is a coexisting iron deficiency, megaloblastic changes in erythroid precursors may not be apparent. Pedersen et al.[322] were the first to describe the ability of the coexisting iron deficiency to partially or completely mask the typical megaloblastic changes in erythroid precursors in pernicious anemia. In some instances of combined iron and nutritional deficiency, modified megaloblasts may be found in the marrow,[157] and the anemia may be dimorphic, with both macroovalocytes and hypochromic microcytes in the peripheral blood. In other cases, despite the deficiency of vitamin B_{12}, the erythroid precursors may appear to be normoblastic or macronormoblastic, and the peripheral blood erythrocytes appear hypochromic and microcytic. After treatment with iron the marrow

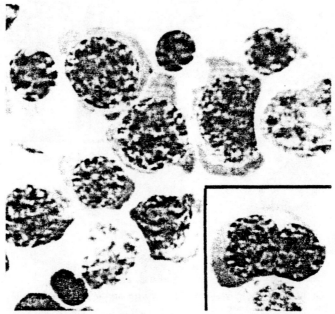

Figure 49. Bone marrow, mild pernicious anemia, illustrating early megaloblastic changes in erythroid precursors. Focal thinning of chromatin strands is observed in some cells, and in others the attenuation of chromatin strands has become more diffuse. Large aggregates of chromatin are seen within the nucleus, and the nucleus has begun to acquire a fenestrated appearance. *Inset:* Multinucleate intermediate megaloblast.

often becomes overtly megaloblastic, and macroovalocytes appear in the peripheral blood, suggesting the underlying nutritional deficiency. In cases of coexisting iron deficiency and vitamin B_{12} or folate deficiency where erythroid precursors do not demonstrate typical megaloblastic changes, the presence of giant metamyelocytes in the marrow and hypersegmented polymorphonuclear leukocytes in the peripheral blood may serve as a diagnostic clue to the possibility of a concomitant deficiency of vitamin B_{12} or folate.

Recent studies have helped to shed light on the mechanisms that enable a coexisting iron deficiency to prevent the development of and thereby camouflage typical megaloblastic changes in pernicious anemia.[408,435] Most of the available evidence to date indicates that iron deficiency causes decreased activity of the iron-dependent ribonucleoside diphosphate reductase, an enzyme responsible for conversion of ribonucleotides to deoxyribonucleotides.[408] In iron deficiency states, decreased activity of this enzyme leads to increased amounts of deoxyuridine monophosphate. The high levels of deoxyuridine monophosphate are converted, presumably by nonenzymatic routes, to thymine DNA, thus enabling the erythroid precursor to appear normoblastic or only mildly megaloblastic rather than markedly megaloblastic. Correction of the iron deficiency[435] apparently leads to

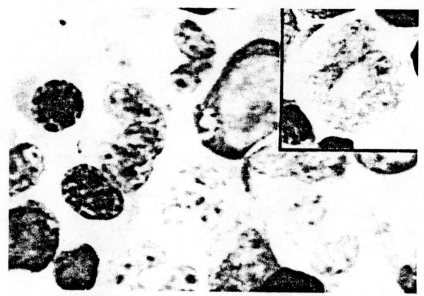

Figure 50. Giant metamyelocytes and bands with atypical twisted nuclei from a patient with mild pernicious anemia.

restoration of the ribonucleoside diphosphate reductase activity and subsequently to decreased amounts of deoxyuridine monophosphate available for conversion into DNA. Under these conditions, the defect in DNA synthesis in vitamin B_{12} deficiency becomes overtly manifest, and the erythroid precursors then appear typically megaloblastic.

Cells of the granulocytic series show abnormalities in patients with mild pernicious anemia. Giant metamyelocytes and bands with clubbed ends of their nuclei and unusual nuclear twistings are found, as are hypersegmented macropolymorphonuclear leukocytes (Fig. 50). Interspersed among these abnormal-appearing granulocyte precursors are myelocytes and metamyelocytes that appear morphologically normal, as are normal-appearing erythroid precursors. It seems as though there is a dual population of both erythroid and granulocyte cells at this stage. Abnormalities in megakaryocytes and plasma cells are usually not observed.

Case III   Moderately Severe Pernicious Anemia

A 51-year-old man was well until one week prior to admission when he developed recurrent hematemesis. On physical examination at the University of Michigan Medical Center his blood pressure was 140/90 mm Hg, and pulse 100 per minute. Pertinent physical findings included slightly decreased sensation to pinprick, vibration, and position sense in both lower extremities. Laboratory test results included a hemoglobin of 9.3 gm%, hematocrit 27%, red blood cell count 2.3 million/mm^3, mean corpuscular volume 119.5 cubic microns, mean corpuscular

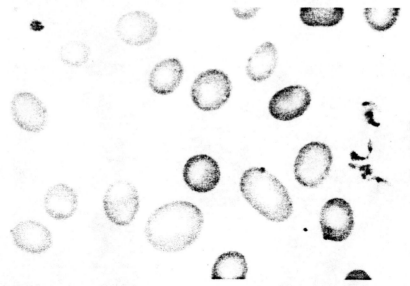

Figure 51. Peripheral blood from a patient with moderate pernicious anemia. Large macroovalocytes and small microcytes are seen, as well as erythrocytes that appear normal in size.

hemoglobin concentration 33.5%, and reticulocyte count 1.1%. The white blood cell count was 3750/mm^3 with 41% polymorphonuclear leukocytes, 14% lymphocytes, 7% monocytes, 35% broken cells, 2% eosinophils, and 1% band forms. The platelet count was 170,000/mm^3. Serum B$_{12}$ was 43 pg/ml, serum folate 10.6 ng/ml, serum iron 60 μg%, LDH 294 units. The Schilling test without intrinsic factor showed 0.28% excretion of radioactivity, and after intrinsic factor the excretion was 14%.

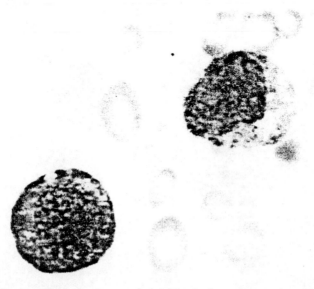

Figure 52. Myelocyte in the peripheral blood of a patient with moderate pernicious anemia. *Inset:* megaloblast, peripheral blood.

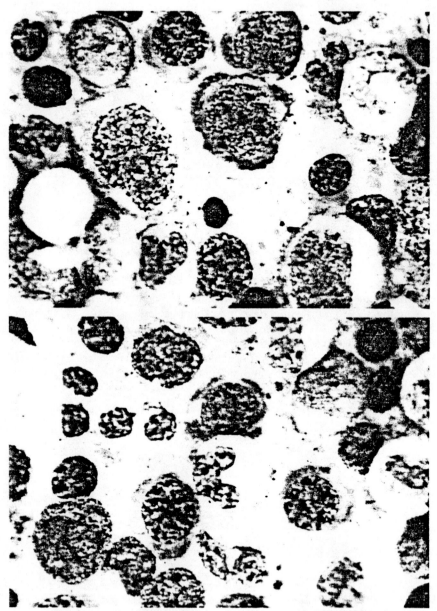

Figure 53.   Bone marrow, moderate pernicious anemia, showing increased numbers of proerythroblasts, giant metamyelocytes, and megaloblasts in various stages of maturation.

The findings of an upper GI series were normal, and gastroscopy did not reveal either bleeding site or obvious gastric atrophy.

The peripheral blood of patients with moderately severe pernicious anemia who have hemoglobin levels between 8.0 and 10.0 grams percent usually shows marked macroovalocytosis (Fig. 51), and the erythrocyte mean corpuscular volume usually exceeds 100 cubic microns. Substantial numbers of microcytes and occasional schistocytes may also be found. Basophilic stippling of erythrocytes may be seen as well. At this stage of the anemia, circulating megaloblasts and proerythroblasts may occasionally be found (Fig. 52). Macropolymorphonuclear leukocytes are commonly observed, and, rarely, myelocytes and metamyelocytes may be seen (Fig. 52).

The bone marrows of patients with pernicious anemia who have hemoglobins between 8.0 and 10.0 grams percent usually show substantial erythroid hyperplasia with increased numbers of proerythroblasts (Fig. 53). Megaloblastic erythropoiesis is found in the majority of the early intermediate and late intermediate megaloblasts (Fig. 53), some of which show coarse cytoplasmic basophilic stippling and multiple Howell-Jolly bodies (Fig. 54).

Degenerating megaloblasts may be seen infrequently (Fig. 54). Erythrophagocytosis by large reticulum cells is also evident. Some of these phagocytes contain degenerating small megaloblasts, mature erythrocytes, and large aggregates of hemosiderin. Megakaryocytes at

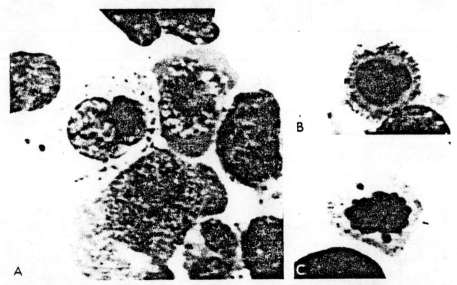

Figure 54. **A.** Coarse cytoplasmic basophilic stippling in late megaloblast (top, left) and degenerating intermediate megaloblast with vacuous-appearing nucleus (top, center). **B.** Degenerating megaloblast with coarse friable-appearing cytoplasm and dense homogeneous nucleus. **C.** Atypical mitotic figure in intermediate megaloblast with coarse cytoplasmic basophilic stippling and Howell-Jolly body in the cytoplasm.

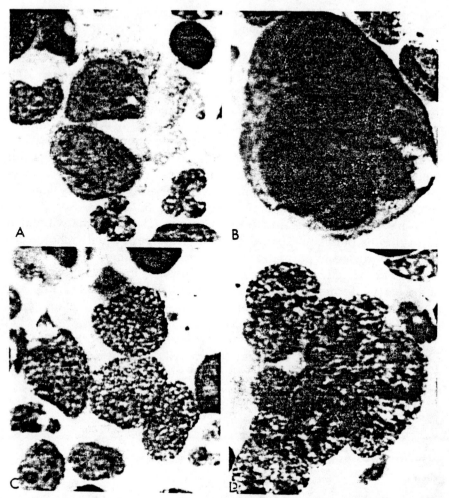

Figure 55. **A.** Megakaryocyte with two nuclei and delicate nuclear chromatin. The cytoplasm is vacuolated and devoid of granules. **B.** Unusually large megakaryocyte with multiple nuclear lobules and basophilic agranular cytoplasm. **C.** Megakaryocyte with unusually coarsely fenestrated chromatin and four separate nuclei. Cytoplasmic granularity is sparse. **D.** Giant megakaryocyte with many nuclear lobulations. The nuclear chromatin is coarse-appearing, and there are scattered large aggregates of chromatin. The cytoplasm is sparsely granular.

this stage of the anemia show abnormalities as illustrated in Figure 55. These megakaryocyte abnormalities include separated nuclear lobes, attenuation of chromatin strands, vacuolization of the cytoplasm, and agranularity of the cytoplasm. Giant metamyelocytes and band forms with serpentine nuclei and bulbous nuclear endings are frequently observed (Fig. 56).

Abnormalities in reticulum cells and hemohistioblasts may also be found. These include large reticulum cells, some of which can be binucleate, and large hemohistioblasts with multiple nucleoli. At

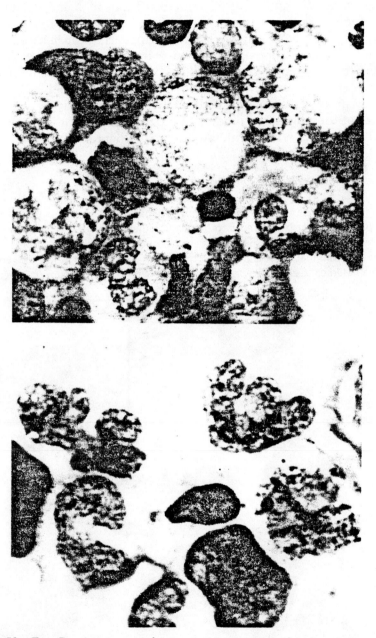

Figure 56. *Top:* Bone marrow, moderate pernicious anemia, showing giant metamyelocytes with twisted nuclei. *Bottom:* Bone marrow, moderate pernicious anemia, illustrating giant metamyelocytes having nuclear lobulations, bulbous ends, and serpentine nuclear configurations.

times, forms that seem to be transitional between hemohistioblasts and erythroid cells (proerythroblasts) can be observed. Whether these represent "erythrogones" as described by Dameshek and Valentine[111] is uncertain.

Increased numbers of both normal-appearing plasma·cells (Fig. 57) and abnormal-appearing plasma cells may be observed at this stage of the anemia. *Mott* or *morula* cells and plasma cells with large, widely separated septa may be seen (Fig. 57). Conceivably, these large plasma cells distended with immunoglobulin may be one of the sources of the plasma antibodies to intrinsic factor and parietal cells found in patients with pernicious anemia (Chapter 10).

Case IV Severe Pernicious Anemia

Six months prior to admission a 49-year-old man noted a progressive weight loss of 15 pounds. He also suffered from dull, nonradiating epigastric pain relieved to some extent by eating food. He noted dyspnea on exertion. Six days prior to admission he was told that he had anemia. On physical examination at the University of Michigan Medical Center he was markedly pale with blood pressure of 120/50 mm

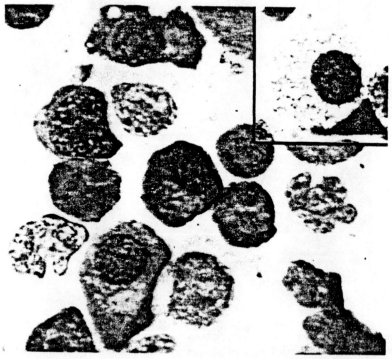

Figure 57.   Increased numbers of mature-appearing plasma cells from bone marrow of patient with moderate pernicious anemia. Several intermediate megaloblasts and hypersegmented polymorphonuclear leukocytes are also seen. *Inset:* aberrant-appearing plasma cell from a patient with moderate pernicious anemia. The cytoplasm of the cell is filled with vacuoles of various sizes, and the nucleus is located eccentrically.

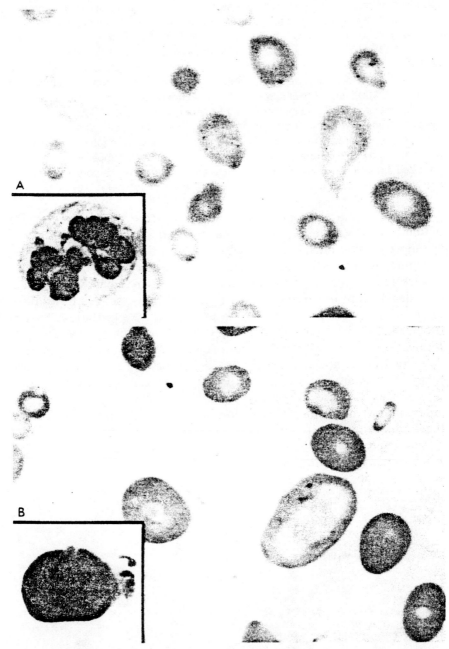

Figure 58. **A.** Peripheral blood from a patient with severe pernicious anemia. Unusually large teardrop poikilocytes, microspherocytes, macroovalocytes, tiny microcytes, thin, pale-appearing elliptocytes and erythrocytes appearing normal in size are observed. *Inset:* giant, hypersegmented polymorphonuclear leukocyte. **B.** Peripheral blood, severe pernicious anemia, showing marked anisopoikilocytosis of erythrocytes, microspherocytes, and a giant macroovalocyte. *Inset:* dwarf megakaryocyte.

Hg, and pulse of 110 per minute. Pertinent physical findings included an atrophic-appearing tongue, grade 3/6 systolic murmur at the cardiac apex, and normal neurological examination. Laboratory test results included a hemoglobin of 5.8 gm%, hematocrit 17.2%, red blood cell count 1.59 million/mm³, mean corpuscular volume 108 cu μ, mean corpuscular hemoglobin concentration 34.6%, and reticulocyte count of 1.8%. The white blood cell count was 2600/mm³ with 73% polymorphonuclear leukocytes, 25% lymphocytes, and 2% eosinophils. The platelet count was 88,000/mm³. Other laboratory data included serum iron of 200 μg%, total iron binding capacity 255 μg%, serum B₁₂ 32 pg/ml, serum folate 7.4 ng/ml, negative direct Coombs' test, serum hemoglobin 2.2 mg%, and LDH 600 units. On gastric analysis, despite proper radiologic placement of the nasogastric tube, no secretions were obtained either before or after histamine stimulation. An upper GI series demonstrated atrophic gastritis, and a Schilling test without intrinsic factor showed 2.4% excretion of radioactivity.

The peripheral blood in cases of severe pernicious anemia in which hemoglobin levels are between 3.0 and 5.0 grams percent show the most marked aniso- and poikilocytosis in the spectrum of the developing severity of anemia in pernicious anemia (Fig. 58). In contrast to less severe forms of the anemia in which macrocytes and macroovalocytes are observed frequently, in the most severe form these large erythrocytes may actually be infrequent. Nevertheless, in untreated cases, large macroovalocytes are always present even if in reduced numbers compared to less severe cases. Numerous tiny microcytes as described originally by Eichhorst[134,135] are observed, and many misshapen erythrocytes or poikilocytes as originally described by Quincke[338-340] are frequently seen. The erythrocyte mean corpuscular volume may sometimes be normal or on occasion low because of these numerous small microcytes and poikilocytes.

Coarse cytoplasmic basophilic stippling of erythrocytes, erythrocytes containing multiple Howell-Jolly bodies (Fig. 59), spherocytes,

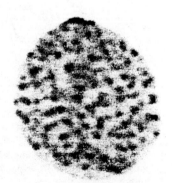 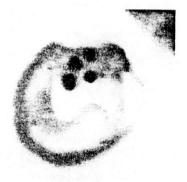

Figure 59. Left: coarse basophilic stippling in erythrocytes. (x 3000 after enlargement.) *Right:* giant macrocyte containing multiple Howell-Jolly bodies. (x 3000 after enlargement.)

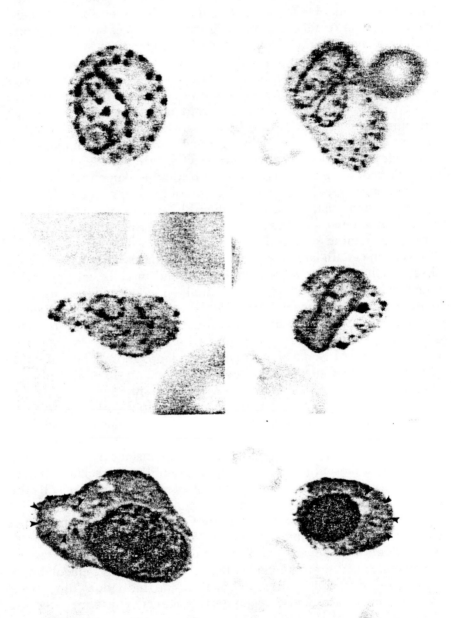

Figure 60. Cabot rings in erythrocytes. Many of the erythrocytes show coarse cytoplasmic basophilic and acidophilic stippling. In some instances, the stippled granules adhere to the Cabot rings, resembling a "necklace." Some of the Cabot rings are oval; others have a figure-eight configuration. (x 3000 after enlargement.) *Bottom:* Cabot rings (arrows) in peripheral blood megaloblasts. (x 2000 after enlargement.)

giant macrocytes, and ring forms as described by Cabot[66] may also be found (Fig. 60). Cabot rings appear bright red when panoptic stains are used, and coarse-appearing red (acidophilic) or blue (basophilic) granules may also be found within the erythrocyte. Some of these granules appear to adhere to the ring structure. Occasionally the ring assumes a figure-eight configuration. In preparations of peripheral blood stained supravitally with brilliant cresyl blue and counterstained with Wright's stain, Cabot rings are not observed in erythrocytes that contain reticulum. This would seem to indicate that the Cabot ring is a product of an erythroid precursor that has lost its reticulum, perhaps within the bone marrow. Although Cabot originally proposed that these bright red rings were nuclear remnants,[66] to date their pathogenesis is uncertain, and they are believed by some to be artifacts or to be composed of mitotic spindle filaments.[42] They are Feulgen-negative, suggesting that they are not composed of DNA.

In the bone marrow and peripheral blood of some patients with pernicious anemia who have numerous Cabot rings in their erythrocytes, red-staining strand-like or loop-shaped structures can also be observed in certain late intermediate megaloblasts.[247] Isaacs[225] in 1938 observed that "Cabot rings have been found in cells with perfectly intact nuclei and entirely separate from the nuclei," and he illustrated a late intermediate megaloblast containing a Cabot ring. Tsamboulas and Malikiosis[104] also described and illustrated an erythroid precursor containing a Cabot ring in a patient who had typhus. As shown in Figures 60 and 61, some of the strands and loops show continuity with either the nuclear membrane or nuclear chromatin. In other cells, the strands and loops appear "free" in the cytoplasm.

Strands and loops such as these are most frequently observed in late megaloblasts that have unusually coarse cytoplasmic basophilic and acidophilic stippling, and frequently their nuclei appear disrupted and perhaps degenerating. In some instances, the coarsely stippled granules adhere to the loops, resembling a necklace. These red-staining strands and loops in certain late megaloblasts may be the precursors of or actual Cabot rings.

Recently, certain properties of the Cabot ring have been studied using various cytochemical reagents.[247] Peripheral blood films from two patients with severe pernicious anemia who had Cabot rings in peripheral blood erythrocytes and in peripheral blood megaloblasts were fixed in acetate-buffered formalin, and individual films were stained with a variety of cytochemical reagents. These included the Feulgen stain to demonstrate DNA, methyl green-pyronin stain to demonstrate both DNA and RNA, Heidenhain's iron hematoxylin stain to visualize mitotic spindle filaments, periodic acid-Schiff (PAS) stain for glycogen, toluidine blue stain for metachromatic substances, alkaline-fast green stain for histones, ammoniacal silver stain to differentiate between lysine-rich and arginine-rich histones, and Prussian blue reagent for iron in conjunction with neutral red counterstain.

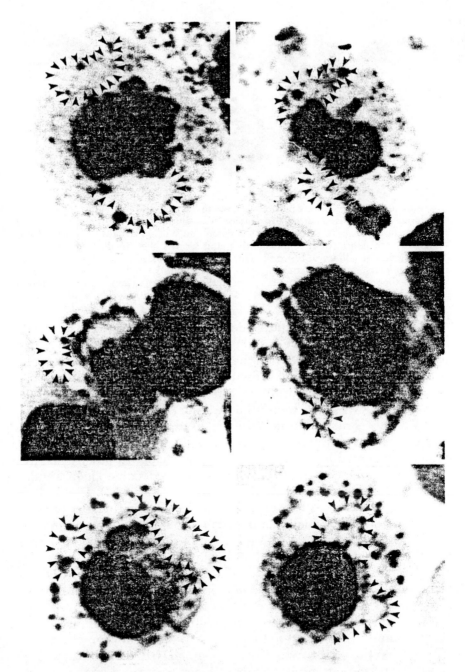

Figure 61. Late intermediate megaloblasts, bone marrow, pernicious anemia. These cells have coarse basophilic and acidophilic stippling and red strands and loops in the cytoplasm (arrows). Some of the strands and loops appear to show continuity with the nuclear membrane or nuclear chromatin. Other strands and loops are located in the cytoplasm in close proximity to the coarse granules. These strands and loops appear most frequently in late megaloblasts that show unusually coarse cytoplasmic basophilic and acidophilic stippling. In many instances the stippled granules adhere to the strands or loops, resembling those seen in typical Cabot rings. These strands and loops in late megaloblasts may be the precursors of or actual Cabot rings.

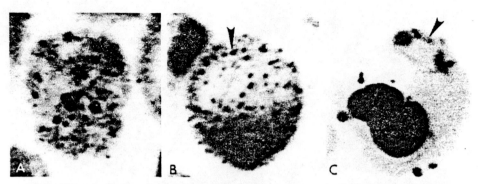

Figure 62. **A.** Figure-eight shaped Cabot ring in ammoniacal silver-stained erythrocyte. Brown and black-staining particles adhere to the ring, and some appear free in the cytoplasm. **B.** Cabot ring (arrow) in ammoniacal silver-stained erythrocyte. **C.** Late intermediate megaloblast stained with Prussian-blue stain to visualize iron and counterstained with neutral red. A red-staining ring form is seen in the cytoplasm, and siderotic granules adhere to the ring. This apparent "necklace" of siderotic granules may be a precursor of or an actual Cabot ring and suggests that the Cabot ring may be related to abnormalities in iron metabolism in those instances where it is composed of both a red strand and coarsely stippled granules (presumably siderotic granules).

These cytochemical studies demonstrated a green ring to which green-staining particles were sometimes attached when the alkaline-fast green stain was used. When the ammoniacal silver stain was used, the ring structure stained brown or black, and coarse-appearing orange and deep yellow or brown particles were observed randomly in the erythrocyte and adherent to the ring (Figs. 62A and 62B).

When the Prussian blue stain was used, erythrocytes containing coarse siderotic granules were observed. In some of these cells, the granules appeared to be arranged in a ring shape. In other cells, the siderotic granules seemed to be adherent to a red-stained loop, similar to that seen in marrow erythroid precursors (Fig. 62C). In all other cytochemical tests, structures analogous to Cabot rings as demonstrated with conventional panoptic stains could not be observed.

Recent ultrastructural studies of Cabot rings were made possible by the unique affinity of the Cabot ring for the ammoniacal silver stain and the high electron density of silver. Electron micrographs of ammoniacal silver stained erythrocytes containing Cabot rings are shown in Figure 63. Dense deposits of silver in a partial ring, loop, serpentine, or figure-eight form were observed in ultrathin sections. Small silver granules were scattered randomly in the cytoplasm of erythrocytes. When the erythrocyte was post-stained with uranyl magnesium acetate and lead citrate, no "matrix"-type structure or structures resembling mitotic spindle filaments could be observed underlying the silver grains in the Cabot ring.

On the basis of these cytochemical studies, it appeared as though one of the constituents of the Cabot ring was histone. The brown black color of the ring as demonstrated by the ammoniacal silver stain suggested that the histone may be arginine-rich. The granular portion

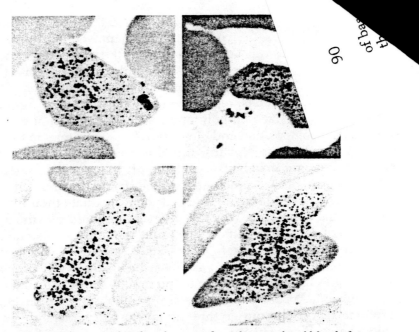

Figure 63. Electron micrographs of erythrocytes from the peripheral blood of a patient with severe pernicious anemia. Many of the patient's erythrocytes contained Cabot rings. A suspension of heparinized peripheral blood containing these cells was fixed in acetate-buffered formalin, stained with the ammoniacal silver reagent, imbedded in Epon, sectioned, and post-stained with uranyl magnesium acetate and lead citrate. Coarse-appearing silver granules indicating the localization of arginine-rich histone are seen in partial ring, loop, serpentine, or figure-eight forms. Occasional small silver grains are scattered randomly throughout the cytoplasm of the erythrocyte. (x 10,000.)

of the ring appeared to be composed of both histone and nonhemo-globin iron. Notably, structures resembling Cabot rings were not observed either with the Feulgen stain or with the methyl green stain, indicating that the Cabot rings probably did not contain DNA. The ultrastructural study of Cabot rings also supports the viewpoint that DNA is not an observable component of the ring. Because uranyl magnesium acetate and lead citrate preferentially stain nucleic acids, the inability to visualize a "matrix" underlying the silver grains suggests that, by this procedure, DNA is either not present in the Cabot ring or may be present in amounts too small to be detected.

Although these studies provide insight into the composition of the Cabot ring, the mechanisms by which nonhemoglobin iron, arginine-rich histone, and perhaps other as yet unidentified substances become associated to form the ring can only be speculated upon at this point. Granules that are identified as coarse basophilic stippling often contain iron.[244] These granules may be found in refractory sideroblastic anemias, and their presence in these anemias as well as in pernicious anemia is believed to represent cytological evidence for disturbed iron metabolism.[244] Consequently, the presence

ophilic stippled granules in and around the Cabot ring suggests
that abnormalities in iron metabolism may contribute to the
pathogenesis of the ring. In other instances the granular portion of the
Cabot ring may be composed of acidophilic stippled granules, and
thus far their composition is undetermined.

In terms of histones, recent evidence indicates that arginine-rich
histone is synthesized on polysomes in the cytoplasm of cells[348] and
that histone composition and biosynthesis are abnormal in pernicious
anemia megaloblasts.[240] Thus, the abnormalities of histone biosynthesis[240] and iron metabolism (Chapter 10) that occur in pernicious
anemia megaloblasts, combined with the spatial proximity of iron and
histone in the cytoplasm of these cells, may facilitate their interaction
to create the Cabot ring. Why this interaction should take the form of a
loop or figure-eight is unknown. Possibly the iron and histone assume
a ring form as the result of "cytoplasmic currents"[42] within the erythroid precursor. Although they have been described primarily in
erythrocytes in pernicious anemia and in some cases of lead poisoning
and leukemia,[66] Cabot rings have also been observed occasionally in
erythrocytes in chronic erythremic myelosis[244] and rarely in erythroleukemia (Chapter 10).

Megaloblasts may also be observed in the peripheral blood (Fig.
64), and occasionally mitotic figures in erythroid precursors may be
found (Fig. 64, inset). The degree of megaloblastemia does not seem
to be related to the degree of anemia, and in severe cases of pernicious
anemia, megaloblastemia is not always observed. At times, erythroid

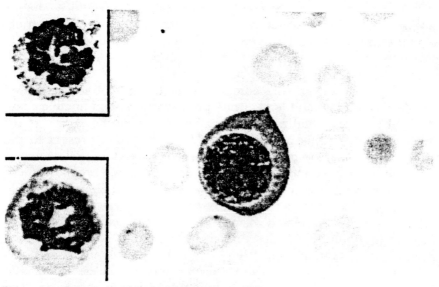

Figure 64. Intermediate megaloblast in the peripheral blood of a patient with severe
pernicious anemia. *Insets:* mitotic figures in megaloblasts, peripheral blood.

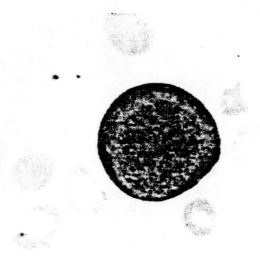

Figure 65. Proerythroblast from the peripheral blood of a patient with severe pernicious anemia.

precursors as young as proerythroblasts may be found in the peripheral blood (Fig. 65). Factors contributing to the release of megaloblasts from the bone marrow and their emergence into the peripheral blood are not as yet understood.

Hypersegmented macropolymorphonuclear leukocytes are frequently observed. In severe pernicious anemia, some of these cells are unusually large and may have as many as 12 to 15 nuclear lobulations (Fig. 58A). The total white blood cell count is usually reduced, and leukopenia as low as 1000 white blood cells per cubic millimeter may be found at this stage of the anemia. Lymphocytes and monocytes may also appear large and aberrant, with loosening and attenuation of nuclear chromatin and multiple lobulations of the monocyte nucleus. Progranulocytes, myelocytes, and aberrant-appearing metamyelocytes and bands may also be found (Fig. 66). Platelets are usually markedly reduced in number, and, occasionally, dwarf megakaryocytes are seen (Fig. 58B).

In cases of severe pernicious anemia with hemoglobin levels between 3.0 and 5.0 grams percent, the most pronounced changes in erythroid and granulocytic precursors may be observed in the bone marrow. Striking erythroid hyperplasia is seen, and proerythroblasts are usually markedly increased in number (Figs. 67 and 68).

Marked megaloblastic changes are seen in virtually all of the erythroid precursors beyond the proerythroblast stage (Figs. 67 and 68). The majority of the erythroid precursors are early and late inter-

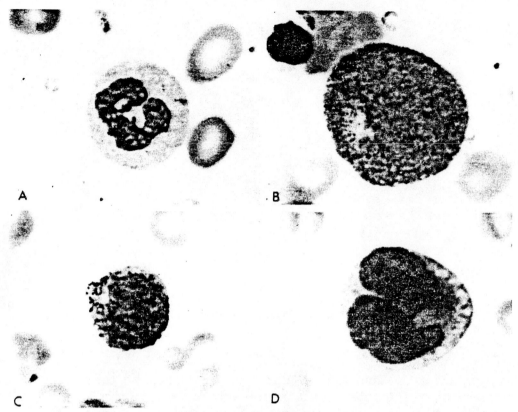

Figure 66. **A.** Large aberrant-appearing polymorphonuclear leukocyte; **B.** large myelocyte in the peripheral blood; **C.** myelocyte with unusually coarse-appearing basophilic granulation from the peripheral blood of a patient with severe pernicious anemia; **D.** monocyte, peripheral blood, showing aberrant nuclear configuration and delicate-appearing nuclear chromatin.

mediate megaloblasts, and chromatin aggregates in their nuclei are scarce.

Increased numbers of mitotic figures in erythroid precursors are frequently observed, and at times these mitotic figures appear aberrant (Fig. 69). Thin, elongated chromosomes such as those described by Powsner and Berman[331] may be seen in some of these mitotic figures, and twisting and intertwining of chromosomes are prominent findings. Factors responsible for these chromosomal aberrations are not well understood but may be related to abnormalities in the biosynthesis of DNA and histone (Chapter 10).

Howell-Jolly bodies are often found in early and late intermediate megaloblasts, particularly in cases of more severe pernicious anemia. These structures are spherical and often vary in size. They contain DNA, are Feulgen-positive, and may appear refractile under the phase contrast microscope. Although small, single Howell-Jolly bodies may be found in erythroid precursors in normal bone marrows, multiple Howell-Jolly bodies within the same cell are usually found only in disorders of erythropoiesis, particularly nutritional megaloblastic anemias and certain primary acquired refractory anemias.[241,244]

There may be several mechanisms responsible for the pathogenesis of Howell-Jolly bodies in pernicious anemia megaloblasts. The first of these has been called abnormal karyorrhexis, in which it is believed that particles of chromosomes fail to unite with the nuclear

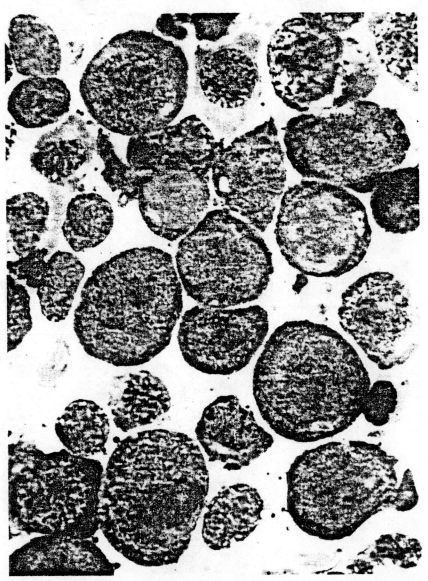

Figure 67. Bone marrow, severe pernicious anemia, showing markedly increased numbers of proerythroblasts. Megaloblasts in various stages of maturation and degeneration are also seen.

chromatin during abnormal mitotic divisions.[42,117,224] These *free* fragments of chromosomes appear as Howell-Jolly bodies in the cytoplasm of the erythroid precursor. An example of abnormal karyorrhexis with isolated chromosomal fragments is shown in Figure 69, upper right.

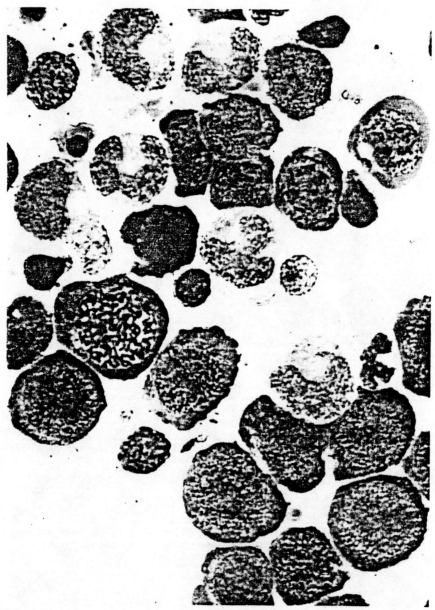

Figure 68. Bone marrow, severe pernicious anemia, showing hyperplasia of proerythroblasts and intermediate megaloblasts, and increased numbers of giant metamyelocytes and bands.

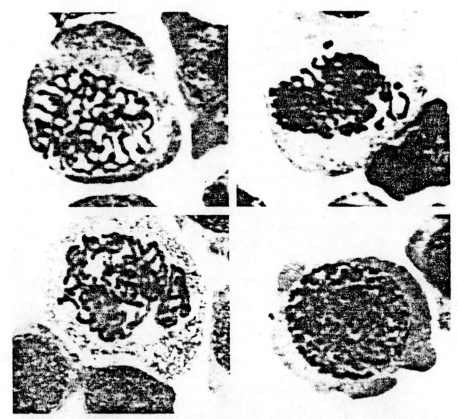

Figure 69. Aberrant mitotic figures in erythroid precursors, bone marrow, severe pernicious anemia. The chromosomes appear unusually long and twisted. Occasionally fragments of chromatin unattached to chromosomes may be observed isolated in the cytoplasm (top right). This phenomenon is known as abnormal karyorrhexis.

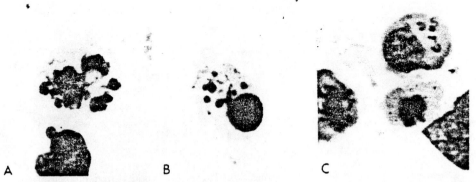

A   B   C

Figure 70. *A.* Degenerating late megaloblast with multiple Howell-Jolly bodies connected to the main nucleus by delicate threads of chromatin. *B.* Degenerating late megaloblast with pyknotic nucleus, multiple Howell-Jolly bodies, and nuclear filaments. *C.* Late intermediate megaloblast (upper right) with several comma-shaped inclusions in the cytoplasm. These inclusions may be Pappenheimer bodies or unusually shaped filaments of chromatin.

A second mechanism for the formation of Howell-Jolly bodies in pernicious anemia is shown in Figure 70. In this process there is an abnormal acceleration of pyknosis, leading to bizarre-appearing multiple nuclear lobulations connected by filamentous strands to a dense-appearing mass of chromatin. Subsequent detachment of these nuclear lobules resulting from abnormal pyknosis is believed to lead to the formation of Howell-Jolly bodies.[42] Examples of these unusually shaped pyknotic nuclei are seen in Figure 70. Comma or coccoid-shaped inclusions, perhaps representing either twisted strands of chromatin or Pappenheimer bodies, may also be found in the cytoplasm of certain late intermediate megaloblasts in pernicious anemia (Fig. 70).

Figure 71 illustrates what may be a third mechanism for the pathogenesis of Howell-Jolly bodies in pernicious anemia. In Figure 71A, a small bleb is seen on the surface of the nuclear membrane of an intermediate megaloblast. Actual "pinching off" of these blebs to form Howell-Jolly bodies has been observed by Lessin and Bessis in

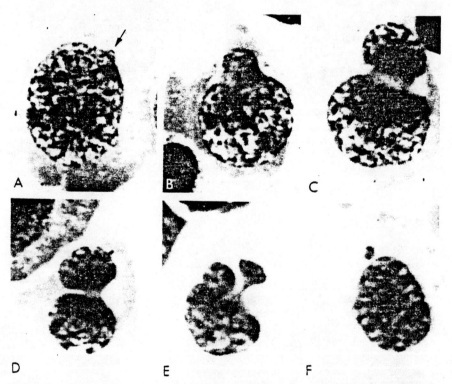

Figure 71.   Proposed sequential formation of Howell-Jolly bodies from nuclear blebs. *A.* Small nuclear bleb (arrow) in megaloblast. *B.* Early enlargement of bleb. *C.* Progressive enlargement of bleb, now filled with substantial amounts of nucleoplasm. *D.* Area of constriction between bleb and main nucleus has intensified. *E.* Bleb connected to main nucleus by thin thread of nucleoplasm. *F.* Free Howell-Jolly body in the cytoplasm, presumably having detached from the main nucleus by severance of the thin connection shown in E.

phase contrast preparations of living megaloblasts.[271] In some instances, multiple nuclear blebs may be seen, and presumably they could give rise to multiple Howell-Jolly bodies by the mechanism described. A proposed sequence of Howell-Jolly body formation by progressive enlargement of this nuclear bleb is shown in Figure 71. In one of these photomicrographs, the enlarged bleb containing nucleoplasm is connected to the main nucleus by a thread-like strand of chromatin. Separation of this connection with the main nucleus may then result in the formation of a free knob-shaped structure (Howell-Jolly body) within the cytoplasm.[42] To date, factors responsible for localized outpouching of the nuclear membrane in the form of blebs are unknown.

The nuclear bleb may also be the precursor of a binucleate proerythroblast or megaloblast by enlarging progressively and ac-

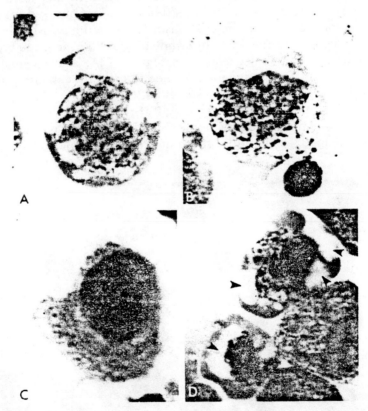

Figure 72. A. Degenerating megaloblast showing multiple large cytoplasmic vacuoles and thinning of nuclear chromatin. B. Degenerating megaloblast demonstrating areas of the nucleus that are virtually devoid of nuclear chromatin. C. Degenerating megaloblast with dense, homogeneous-appearing nucleus and ragged cytoplasm. D. Megaloblasts containing eosinophilic-staining oval-shaped areas in the cytoplasm, presumably representing sequestrations of hemoglobin (arrows). These areas are separated by deeply basophilic cytoplasm. Cells such as these provide cytological evidence for defective hemoglobinization of megaloblasts in pernicious anemia.

commodating large quantities of nucleoplasm and then separating from the main nucleus (Fig. 71). Multinucleate megaloblasts may also arise as a result of asynchronous and abnormal nuclear divisions.[41,365,369]

Frequently there are unusual morphological abnormalities of intermediate megaloblaasts in the bone marrow of patients with severe untreated pernicious anemia.[246] Some of these abnormalities may reflect degenerative changes whereas others may represent abnormalities of hemoglobinization. In Figures 72A, B, and C, three types of degenerating megaloblasts are illustrated. In Figure 72A the megaloblast demonstrates multiple large cytoplasmic vacuoles. In Figure 72B the megaloblast nucleus has unusually marked fenestration of the chromatin pattern and in some areas the nucleus seems to be virtually devoid of chromatin. Similar vacuous nuclear chromatin areas may be seen in the nucleus of the megaloblast in Figure 72A. Figure 72C depicts a third type of degenerating megaloblast. In this cell the nuclear chromatin has lost its fine detail and appears dense and homogeneous. Likewise, the cytoplasm of this cell has lost detail and appears ragged with frayed cytoplasmic borders. These three types of degenerating megaloblasts shown in Figures 72A, B, and C may constitute cytological evidence for intramedullary cell death and ineffective erythropoiesis in pernicious anemia.[246]

A fourth type of unusual abnormality of megaloblasts in untreated pernicious anemia is seen in Figure 72D. In these megaloblasts there are oval-shaped eosinophilic-staining areas, presumably containing

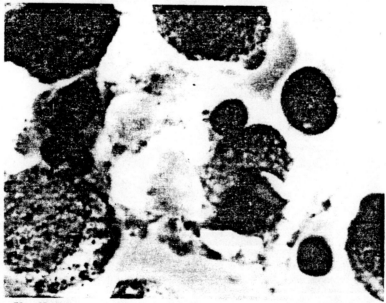

Figure 73. Histiocyte containing erythrocyte and partially degraded erythroid precursors in the cytoplasm.

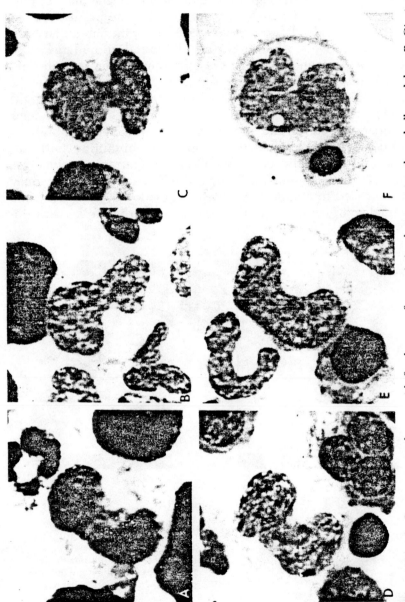

Figure 74. *A.* Giant metamyelocyte with focal areas of constriction between two large bulbous lobes. *B.* Giant metamyelocytes with unusually large and bulbous nuclear end. *C.* Giant metamyelocyte with dumbbell-shaped nucleus. *D-F.* Giant metamyelocytes with squared nuclear configurations. As seen in D, the nuclear endings may appear bulbous, and there may be focal areas of constriction at the right angle bendings of the nucleus, as seen in F.

hemoglobin, alternating with and separated by areas of intensely basophilic cytoplasm that impart an appearance of uneven hemoglobinization to the cell. This apparent sequestration of hemoglobin-containing areas within the cytoplasm may be cytological evidence for a serious defect in the hemoglobinization of the megaloblast in pernicious anemia, and cells such as these may also be predisposed to intramedullary cell death. Additional evidence for intramedullary cell death and ineffective erythropoiesis may be found in the large numbers of histiocytes containing mature erythrocytes and partially degraded megaloblasts in their cytoplasm (Fig. 73).

Granulocytes exhibit marked changes with numerous giant metamyelocytes and bands showing twistings and loopings of their nuclei, square-appearing and serpentine nuclei, nuclei with bulbous ends, and metamyelocytes with cytoplasms containing both eosinophilic and basophilic granulation. These aberrant granulocytes are seen in Figures 74 and 75. Progranulocytes and myelocytes may also be increased in number, but usually they do not show the same type of nuclear or cytoplasmic aberrations as seen in the metamyelocyte.

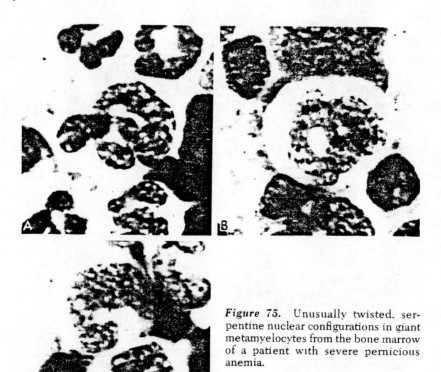

Figure 75.   Unusually twisted, serpentine nuclear configurations in giant metamyelocytes from the bone marrow of a patient with severe pernicious anemia.

Megakaryocytes show abnormalities as seen in Figure 55, and at this stage of the anemia, the megakaryocytes and the peripheral platelet counts are usually markedly reduced in number. Degenerating megakaryocytes with loss of nuclear and cytoplasmic detail may be found. Abnormalities in plasma cells are frequently seen (Fig. 76).

In the bone marrow of patients with severe pernicious anemia, there are often increased numbers of eosinophils, particularly eosinophil myelocytes. As noted earlier, peripheral blood eosinophilia was noted in pernicious anemia by Levine and Ladd[273] in 1921. The significance of the eosinophilia is unknown. Although it has been thought that marrow eosinophilia is more prominent in vitamin B_{12} deficiency than in folate deficiency, it is not possible to distinguish between the two deficiency states with certainty on the basis of a bone marrow examination alone since the megaloblastosis in both conditions is identical.

Sections of clotted bone marrow from patients with severe pernicious anemia show erythroid hyperplasia and increased numbers of large primitive-appearing cells, presumably proerythroblasts and early intermediate megaloblasts. Granulocytic precursors appear en-

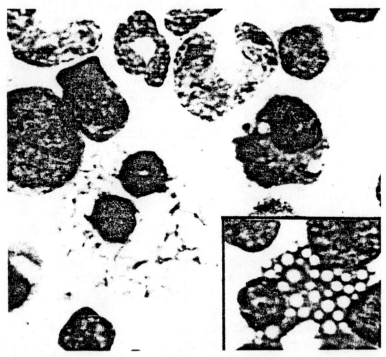

Figure 76. Large, binucleate aberrant-appearing plasma cell containing numerous large distended vacuoles in the cytoplasm (Mott cell). A normal-appearing plasma cell is located to the upper right of this large atypical plasma cell. *Inset:* aberrant plasma cell containing large eosinophilic-staining inclusions (Russell bodies) from the bone marrow of a patient with severe pernicious anemia.

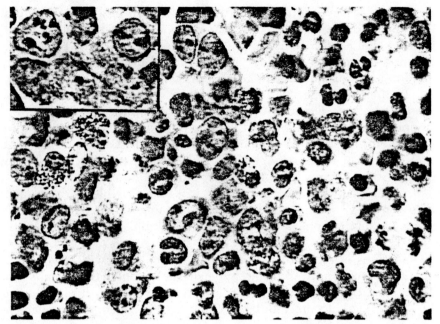

Figure 77. Section of clotted bone marrow, severe pernicious anemia, stained with hematoxylin and eosin. Cells with large, pale vesicular-appearing nuclei and prominent nucleoli represent large proerythroblasts and early intermediate megaloblasts. Erythroid precursors at various stages of maturation and giant granulocytes may also be seen. Inset shows a group of proerythroblasts and megaloblasts.

larged, and eosinophil myelocytes may be increased in number (Fig. 77). A 1-micron thick section of bone marrow from patients with untreated pernicious anemia, fixed in glutaraldehyde imbedded in Epon and stained with lead citrate and uranyl magnesium acetate is shown in Figure 78. Cells with pale vesicular nuclei and prominent nucleoli represent large proerythroblasts and early intermediate megaloblasts. Large granulocytic precursors, late megaloblasts with hyperchromatic nuclei, and several mitotic figures are also observed. Erythroid hyperplasia is seen.

Thin sections of pernicious anemia marrows processed for electron microscopy and examined in collaboration with Dr. Robert H. Gray are seen in Figures 79 to 86. Figure 79 illustrates several large proerythroblasts. The nuclear chromatin is finely dispersed (euchromatin) and shows few if any aggregates of heterochromatin. The cytoplasm contains substantial amounts of rough endoplasmic reticulum and many mitochondria.

A maturational sequence of megaloblasts viewed ultrastructurally is shown in Figures 79 to 81 and Figure 84. Figures 80 and 81 demonstrate early intermediate megaloblasts. Few aggregates of heterochromatin are present in the nucleus, and some of these aggregates appear to be adhering to the nuclear membrane. The cytoplasmic staining appears darker, due to increased content of hemoglobin.

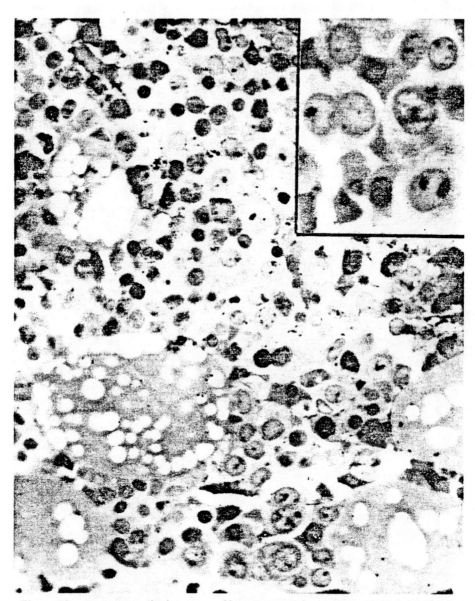

Figure 78. One-micron thick section of bone marrow from patient with severe pernicious anemia fixed in glutaraldehyde and stained with toluidine blue. Large primitive-appearing cells with pale vesicular nuclei and prominent nuclei are proerythroblasts and early intermediate megaloblasts. Other developing megaloblasts at various stages of maturation can be found, as well as large granulocyte precursors. Large fatty globules may also be seen. *Inset:* higher power view of megaloblasts.

Nuclear blebs similar to those found in light micrographs of early intermediate megaloblasts were also observed ultrastructurally (Fig. 82) and appeared to contain nucleoplasm consisting primarily of euchromatin that seemed to become progressively darker and more homogeneous in appearance in more mature megaloblasts (Fig. 83). In some instances the bleb appeared to be partially detached from the nucleus (Fig. 83). Nuclear blebs have also been observed ultrastruc-

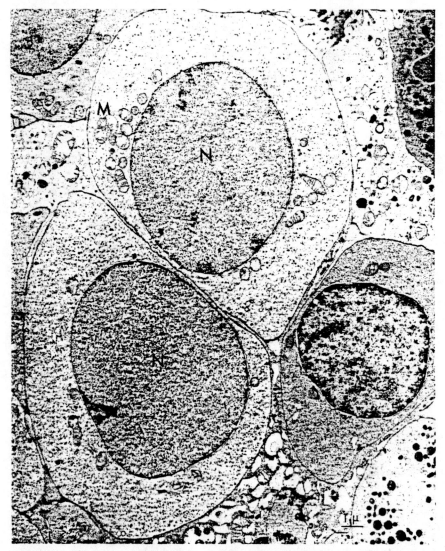

Figure 79. Electron micrograph of two large proerythroblasts from bone marrow of patient with pernicious anemia. The nuclear chromatin appears finely dispersed, and mitochondria and rough endoplasmic reticulum are prominent in the cytoplasm. A smaller late intermediate megaloblast is also seen in the micrograph (middle, right). N = Nucleus, M = Mitochondrion. (x 7500.)

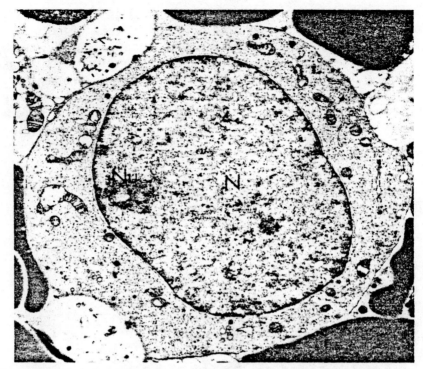

Figure 80.   Electron micrograph of an early intermediate megaloblast showing prominent nucleolus and small amounts of heterochromatin adjacent to and presumably
adherent to the nuclear membrane. Nu = Nucleolus, N = Nucleus. (x 7500.)

turally in erythroid precursors in the DiGuglielmo syndrome[244] and in
leukemic blasts.[42] As mentioned earlier, the budding of blebs from the
nuclear membrane of megaloblasts may be one of the factors responsible for the formation of Howell-Jolly bodies (Fig. 83).

Late intermediate megaloblasts show additional condensation of
nuclear chromatin with considerable amounts of finely dispersed
chromatin interspersed between the aggregates. Some of the late
megaloblasts show aberrant nuclear configurations, as illustrated in
Figure 84. Giant metamyelocytes and bands are also observed, as
depicted in Figure 85. Their nuclei are often folded and twisted and
frequently have bulbous nuclear endings resembling those seen in
the light micrographs. Plasma cells are frequently seen and may contain large vacuoles. Macrophages are increased in number and may
contain vacuoles, cellular debris, and erythrocytes within their cytoplasm (Fig. 86). After treatment with vitamin B_{12}, increased amounts
of heterochromatin are observed in erythroid precursors.[367]

Tables 1 and 2 enumerate various erythroid and granulocytic
morphological abnormalities in pernicious anemia.[241] Most of these
abnormalities may also be found in severe folate deficiency as well as
in pernicious anemia. Because they are found so frequently in nutri-

tional megaloblastic anemias, they are often a diagnostic aid in distinguishing nutritional anemias from refractory anemias of the DiGuglielmo syndrome. At times, these refractory anemias characterized by erythroid hyperplasia and megaloblastoid erythropoiesis[244] have been diagnosed initially as nutritional megaloblastic anemias.

Nowadays, the vast majority of patients with pernicious anemia are treated promptly with vitamin B_{12} shortly after diagnosis, and consequently, the morbid anatomy of this disease described so vividly in

Text continued on page 110

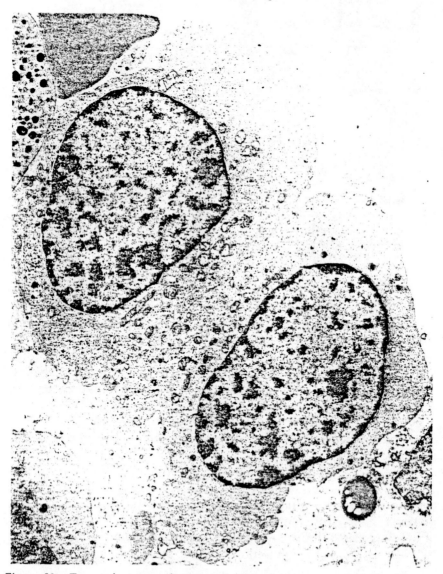

Figure 81. Two early intermediate megaloblasts with greater amounts of heterochromatin than in Figure 80 and substantial amounts of euchromatin. Some of the heterochromatin appears isolated and adherent to the nuclear membrane. (x 7500.)

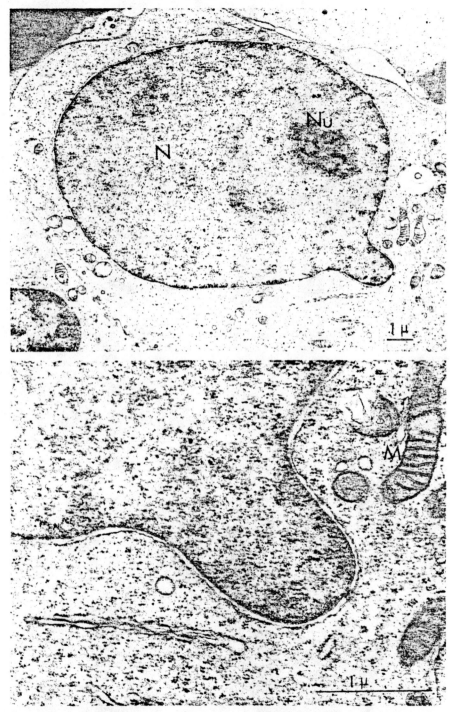

Figure 82. Nuclear bleb in megaloblast (top) and a higher power view of the nuclear bleb containing nucleoplasm (bottom). (Top, x 7500; bottom, x 30,000.)

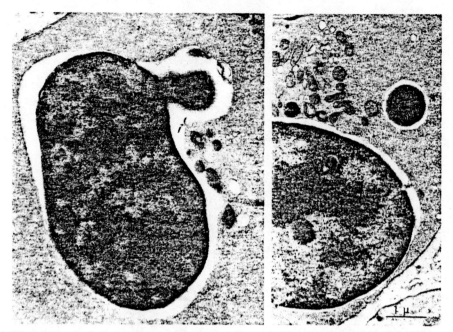

Figure 83. *Left:* large dense-appearing nuclear bleb in a late intermediate megaloblast. An area of constriction between the bleb and the main nucleus can be seen.
(x 15,000.) *Right:* large Howell-Jolly body, presumably arising from severance of the
connection between the dense bleb and the main nucleus. (x 15,000.)

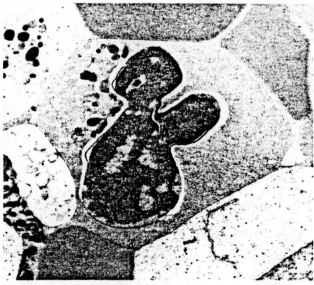

Figure 84. Late intermediate megaloblast with aberrant-appearing cloverleaf nuclear
configuration. (x 7500.)

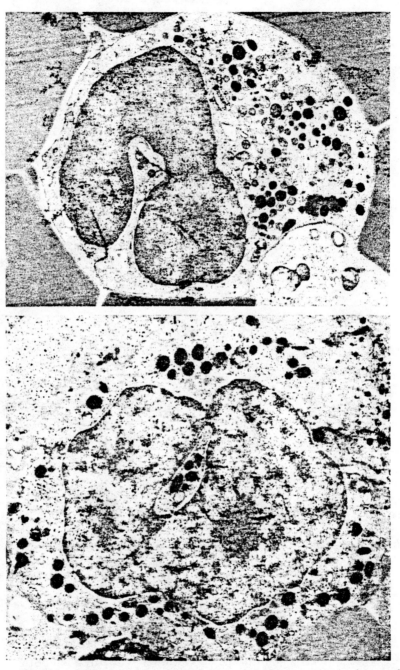

Figure 85.   Two giant metamyelocytes with large aberrant-appearing nuclear configurations and bulbous nuclear endings. (x 7500.)

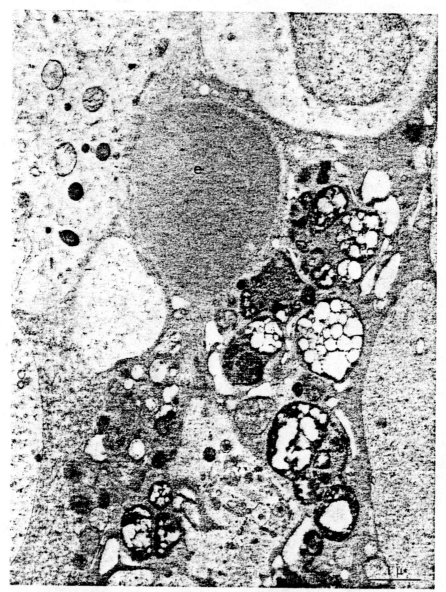

Figure 86. High power view of macrophage cytoplasm showing cellular debris, multiple vacuoles, and an erythrocyte contained within the cytoplasm of the macrophage (erythrophagocytosis). e = erythrocyte. (x 18,000.)

the earlier literature[45,65,218,219,265] is rarely observed. In the past, however, typical necropsy findings in patients who died of pernicious anemia included atrophic gastritis, fatty degenerative changes in visceral organs, particularly the liver and heart, hepatic hemosiderosis and a currant-jelly appearance of the bone marrow which was also found to be heavily laden with iron.

TABLE 1.   *Erythroid Abnormalities in Pernicious Anemia*

Megaloblastic changes are recognized with greatest confidence at the intermediate megaloblastic stage.[241] Proerythroblasts in pernicious anemia cannot be distinguished with assurance from proerythroblasts in a variety of other disorders of erythropoiesis.[241] Although some of these erythroid abnormalities are found most frequently in nutritional megaloblastic anemia, others such as coarse cytoplasmic basophilic stippling may be found in other types of anemia (e.g., DiGuglielmo syndrome, thalassemia) as well.[241,244]

1. Focal attenuation of chromatin strands.
2. Decreased numbers of chromatin aggregates.
3. Fenestration of nuclear chromatin pattern.
4. Nucleocytoplasmic asynchrony.
5. Degenerating megaloblasts with large nuclear areas seemingly devoid of chromatin or nuclei that appear dense and homogeneous. The cytoplasm of these degenerating megaloblasts often appears ragged.[246]
6. Increased numbers of proerythroblasts, some of which are multinucleate.
7. Multiple Howell-Jolly bodies.
8. Nuclear strands.
9. Nuclear blebs.
10. Nuclear *bubbles*.
11. Coarse cytoplasmic basophilic stippling in late intermediate megaloblasts.
12. Unusual coccoid or ring-shaped cytoplasmic inclusions, probably Pappenheimer bodies or Cabot rings.
13. Aberrant-appearing late normoblasts with cloverleaf nuclear chromatin pattern.
14. Aberrant-appearing mitotic figures with thin, elongated chromosomes.
15. Vacuolization of erythroid precursor cytoplasm.
16. Areas of deeply basophilic cytoplasm alternating with areas of eosinophilic-staining material, presumably hemoglobin, within the same cell. This type of morphological abnormality probably represents a severe defect in the hemoglobinization of the megaloblast.[246]

TABLE 2.   *Granulocytic Abnormalities in Pernicious Anemia*

Abnormalities in granulocytic precursors first become recognizable in the early metamyelocyte stage of maturation. Later stages of granulocytic development often show marked abnormalities as well.[241] Reasons why these changes should manifest themselves first morphologically at the metamyelocyte stage are unclear. Although these abnormalities are seen most frequently in nutritional megaloblastic anemia, giant metamyelocytes, bands with doughnut-hole nuclei, and cells containing both eosinophilic and basophilic granulation may also be found in other conditions unassociated with deficiency of vitamin B_{12} or folate, such as acute myeloblastic or myelomonocytic leukemia.

1. Loopings and twistings of the nuclei.
2. Presence of both basophilic and eosinophilic granules in the same cell.
3. Unusual-appearing serpentine nuclei.
4. Nuclei with clubbed or bulbous ends.
5. Hypersegmentation of polymorphonuclear leukocyte nuclei with multiple connections between adjacent nuclear lobes.
6. Square-appearing nuclear configuration of the nucleus of the metamyelocyte with focal constrictions at the right angles of the nuclear bendings.
7. Unusual focal constrictions of the metamyelocyte nucleus.
8. Gigantism of metamyelocytes.
9. Doughnut-hole shaped nuclei.

TREATMENT OF PERNICIOUS ANEMIA

The present-day treatment for pernicious anemia is parenteral vitamin B_{12}.[36,88] At one time, combinations of intrinsic factor and vitamin B_{12} were used orally. Although these combinations were effective in some patients, in others they were found to be ineffective for long-term therapy and have since been abandoned.

Blackburn et al.[48] studied the oral treatment of pernicious anemia with a combined vitamin B_{12} and intrinsic factor preparation. Only 1 of 5 patients had an ineffective response, but this response became satisfactory when the vitamin B_{12} was given parenterally. In 12 patients previously treated by intramuscular vitamin B_{12}, then switched to oral B_{12}-intrinsic factor preparation, the hemoglobin and red blood cell count decreased over one year in 1 patient, and subacute combined degeneration developed.

Berlin et al.[40] found that 22 of 66 cases of pernicious anemia treated with oral vitamin B_{12}-intrinsic factor preparations became refractory to therapy after 12 months. The authors speculated that this refractoriness may have been due to relative differences in the potencies of the intrinsic factor preparations. Waife et al.[412] studied the use of oral vitamin B_{12} without intrinsic factor in the treatment of pernicious anemia. They found that in 27 patients treated with vitamin B_{12} given orally in dosages of 3000 micrograms per day, excellent responses were obtained, and intrinsic factor was not required.

There are a number of satisfactory regimens for the treatment of pernicious anemia.[36,88] One of these programs was developed at the Simpson Memorial Institute and over the years has been found to be effective. It consists of injections of 100 micrograms of vitamin B_{12} daily for seven days, then three times weekly for four weeks, followed by once weekly until erythroid values normalize. Injections of vitamin B_{12} are then continued once every two weeks for one year, then once a month indefinitely. With this treatment program, total replenishment of body vitamin B_{12} stores is believed to occur approximately three years after the initiation of therapy. It should be emphasized that patients with neurological manifestations of vitamin B_{12} deficiency require more intensive treatment with vitamin B_{12} than those with only hematological abnormalities (see Chapter 3).

Parenteral therapy with aqueous liver extract is no longer recommended for the treatment of pernicious anemia, and liver extract is not listed in the *United States Pharmacopeia* at this time. Although hydroxycobalamin is believed to possess certain advantages over cyanocobalamin since it remains in the blood for a longer period of time,[88] in actual practice the hematological response to both agents is indistinguishable.

After initial treatment with vitamin B_{12}, a substantial number of patients with untreated pernicious anemia experience a subjective

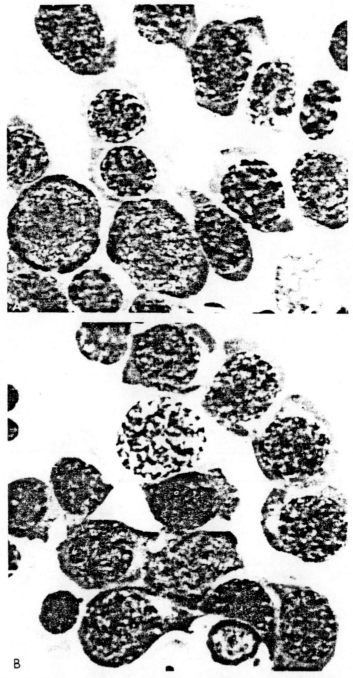

Figure 87. **A.** Bone marrow from a patient with pernicious anemia who had been treated 12 hours earlier with vitamin B_{12}. The erythropoiesis has become macronormoblastic, and hyperplasia of early and late intermediate macronormoblasts may be found. **B.** Bone marrow from a patient with pernicious anemia who had been treated 12 hours earlier with vitamin B_{12}. Early and late intermediate macronormoblasts are intensely basophilic, and occasionally a large megaloblast may be found showing typical nucleocytoplasmic dissociation and fenestrated nuclear chromatin (top, center).

and sometimes dramatic sense of well-being within 8 to 12 hours after receiving the vitamin. In uncomplicated cases the marrow usually becomes macronormoblastic within 8 to 12 hours after administration of vitamin B_{12} (Fig. 87A). Proerythroblasts are usually markedly decreased in number, and the marrow retains its original marked erythroid hyperplasia. However, the majority of the erythroid precursors are early and late intermediate macronormoblasts. A few intermediate megaloblasts may persist, however, and some show evidence of nucleocytoplasmic asynchrony (Fig. 87B). The cytoplasm of the erythroid precursors is deeply basophilic. Some late macronormoblasts continue to exhibit multiple Howell-Jolly bodies.

The rapid changes in the morphological appearance of the erythroid precursors are not paralleled by the granulocytic precursors, however, and giant metamyelocytes and giant band forms may persist in the bone marrow for up to several weeks after therapy. Likewise, hypersegmented polymorphonuclear leukocytes may also remain in the peripheral blood for as long as four to six weeks after the initiation of therapy.

A beginning rise in the number of reticulocytes in the peripheral

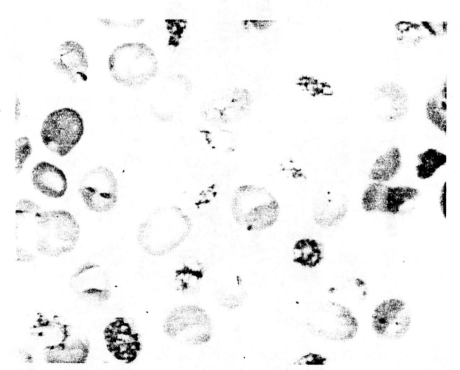

Figure 88. Peripheral blood of a patient with severe pernicious anemia who had been treated 6 days previously with vitamin B_{12}. The photomicrograph of this patient's peripheral blood has been stained supravitally with brilliant cresyl blue to demonstrate the large numbers of reticulocytes.

blood is usually noted on the third or fourth day after therapy is first administered (Fig. 88), as noted originally by Minot and Murphy.[298] The population of reticulocytes is believed to arise from a generation of new erythroid precursors[433] rather than a maturation of reticulocytes from pre-existing megaloblasts. What happens to the megaloblasts after vitamin B_{12} therapy, assuming that they do not mature into reticulocytes is therefore uncertain, but it is believed that many of them undergo intramedullary cell death.[433]

The reticulocyte response usually reaches a peak on the seventh to tenth day. Reticulocyte counts as high as 40% to 50% are usually seen in patients who have unusually low red blood cell counts (1 million per cubic millimeter or less) prior to therapy. Coincident with the rise in reticulocytes, the hemoglobin and hematocrit begin to rise, as do the white blood cell count and platelet count. Approximately 10 days to two weeks after the initial administration of vitamin B_{12}, the reticulocyte count slowly falls. Normalization of erythroid values usually does not occur until four to six weeks after the initiation of therapy. Suboptimal responses to vitamin B_{12} may occur when coincident disorders such as acute or chronic infection, debilitation, or chronic diseases such as rheumatoid arthritis are present.

CHAPTER 3

NEUROLOGICAL COMPLICATIONS OF PERNICIOUS ANEMIA

The neurological complications of vitamin B_{12} deficiency are peripheral neuritis and/or subacute combined degeneration of the spinal cord.[358] The latter is a diffuse disorder, affecting posterior and lateral columns of the spinal cord and may affect the brain as well. Sensory, motor, and psychic changes ensue as a result of the neuropathological lesions. The neurological manifestations of vitamin B_{12} deficiency may precede the appearance of the anemia by months or even years.[88,358] In contrast to the rapid hematological response, the neurological complications of pernicious anemia often show an inconstant and unpredictable response to therapy with vitamin B_{12}.

Historically, Otto Leichtenstern (Fig. 89) in 1884 was the first to

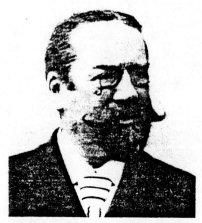

Figure 89. Otto Leichtenstern (1845-1900). (From Galerie hervorragender Aertze und Naturforscher. München. Med. Wschr. 47:430, 1900.)

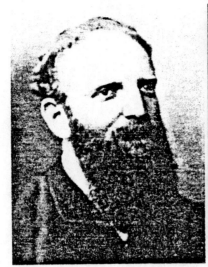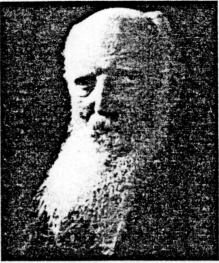

Figure 90. **Left:** Ludwig Lichtheim (1845-1928). (From Schweiz Med. Wschr. *15:527,* 1934. Reproduced by permission of Schwabe & Co., Basel, Switzerland.) **Right:** Lichtheim in later years. (From Schweiz Med. Wschr. 9:226, 1928. Reproduced with permission of Schwabe & Co., Basel, Switzerland.)

describe pernicious anemia in two patients whom he diagnosed as also having tabes dorsalis.[268] Although it was not called such at the time, it is likely that these patients had subacute combined degeneration of the spinal cord as a consequence of vitamin B_{12} deficiency. Leichtenstern noted that there was posterior column degeneration, a feature of so-called combined system disease described earlier in 1878 by Kahler and Pick,[234] but he did not mention sensory changes.

Ludwig Lichtheim (Fig. 90) in 1887 was probably the first to describe accurately subacute combined degeneration of the cord in association with pernicious anemia.[274] Of Lichtheim's three patients with pernicious anemia, one patient had stiffness of the legs, weakness, paresthesias, ataxia, and a positive Romberg sign. There was widespread degeneration of the posterior columns, and foci of degeneration in the lateral and anterior columns, but no demonstrable lesions of the peripheral nerves.

Following Lichtheim's initial report, numerous other reports describing the clinical manifestations and pathology of the spinal cord in cases of pernicious anemia appeared.[46,56,58,60,92,220,265,276,295,334,336,357,418] In 1900, Russell et al.[358] defined the neurological syndrome of pernicious anemia in detail and named it "subacute combined degeneration of the spinal cord." Original figures from their paper of 1900 illustrating the spinal cord lesions and the pattern of sensory loss in one of their patients are reproduced in Figures 91 and 92.

In addition to spinal cord manifestations of vitamin B_{12} deficiency, cerebral manifestations are commonly observed.[70,214,347,374] Camp[70] in 1912 was one of the first to call attention to the mental aberrations

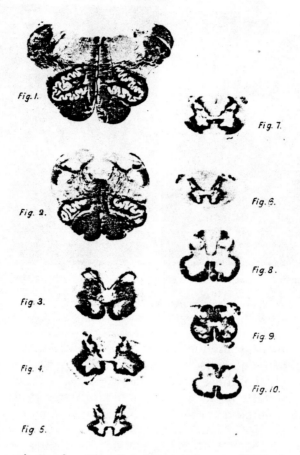

Figure 91. Reproduction from Russell et al.'s original paper of 1900, showing posterior and lateral column degeneration of the spinal cord in patients with neurological conplications of pernicious anemia. (From Brain 23:39, 1900.)

seen in some patients with pernicious anemia. He described a 46-year-old man with pernicious anemia who had mental symptoms resembling those seen in general paresis. According to Holmes et al.[214] these cerebral manifestations include dementia, mood disorders, mental slowness, memory deficit, confusion, severe agitation and depression, delusions, paranoid behavior, visual and auditory hallucinations, urinary and fecal incontinence unrelated to spinal cord lesions, dysphagia, maniacal behavior, and seizures.

One of the most complete early studies of the cerebral pathology of pernicious anemia was made in 1918 by Woltman,[440] who found degenerative areas in the brain similar to those in the cord. These areas were principally in the medulla. Diffuse degeneration was also found in the long tracts, and focal areas of destruction were observed in the gray matter. Adams and Kubik[7] also studied the neuropathological features of cerebral involvement in pernicious anemia. They found diffuse and uneven degeneration of nerve fibers in the spinal

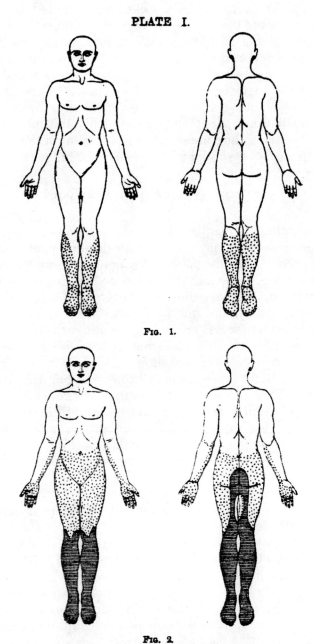

PLATE I.

Fɪɢ. 1.

Fɪɢ. 2.

Fɪɢ. 1.—An early stage in the anæsthesia. Case No. 8.
Fɪɢ. 2.—Anæsthesia early in the flaccid stage. Case No. 4.
(The dotted areas represent partial, the lined areas complete, loss to all forms.)

Figure 92. Plate from Russell et al.'s paper of 1900 showing the typical sensory deficits of subacute combined degeneration of the spinal cord.

cord and the cerebral white matter, with relatively little proliferation of fibrous glia. The cerebral lesions closely resembled those found in the cord, confirming the earlier findings of Woltman.[440]

As a part of the cerebral manifestations, ocular manifestations have been reported as being early and often presenting signs of pernicious anemia. Aside from retinal hemorrhages as reported originally by Biermer[45] and subsequently by MacKenzie,[282] optic atrophy was described by Cohen[93] in 1936 and others[106,235] as being an early manifestation of vitamin B_{12} deficiency. Presumably, the optic atrophy and consequent visual failure are due to involvement of the optic nerves and tracts by a process similar to that seen in the brain and spinal cord.

CLINICAL MANIFESTATIONS

The neurological manifestations of pernicious anemia are often insidious in onset and may precede the development of anemia by months or years. At first the patient may notice numbness and tingling of the extremities, especially in the toes. The fingers may later be involved with similar paresthesias. These paresthesias often spread slowly up the lower limbs and the upper limbs and may involve the trunk. Weakness and ataxia are usually found in the lower limbs and develop generally after the paresthesias have become established. Unusually sharp or stabbing sensations may occur. In the periphery of the extremities, light touch, heat and cold, and pinprick sensibilities are impaired. This ultimately leads to the "stocking and glove" sensory loss distribution as noted by Russell et al.[357,358] Position sense and vibratory sense are impaired in the lower limbs at first and subsequently in the upper limbs. Muscular wasting may be seen in peripheral limb muscles, as well as ataxia, ataxic gait, and Romberg's sign.

Ankle jerks are absent in many patients at the time of diagnosis. Knee jerks are less frequently lost. Rarely the reflexes may be exaggerated. Plantar reflexes are flexor in most cases, but eventually become extensor in almost all. Sphincter disturbances, impotence, and anosmia also may be seen. Pleocytosis of the spinal fluid is usually not observed. Spinal fluid vitamin B_{12} levels are low.

The following is a representative case of subacute combined degeneration of the cord in a patient with pernicious anemia. This patient also had carcinoma of the stomach, a disorder that occurs with increased frequency in patients with pernicious anemia as noted originally by Eisenlohr in 1877.[136]

Case V

Fifteen years prior to admission, a 61-year-old woman was diagnosed as having pernicious anemia. Although she was advised to take regular injections of vitamin

B$_{12}$, she did not do so until several months prior to admission when she began to receive injections of liver extract. Three months prior to admission she developed burning left upper quadrant pain, constipation, and noted a 20-pound weight loss. She also noted depression, anorexia, and insomnia. For 14 years prior to admission she walked with crutches, and noted progressive inability to walk for several months prior to admission.

On physical examination she was an obese, confused woman with blood pressure 130/70 mm Hg, and pulse 60 per minute. Pertinent physical findings included normal funduscopic examination, crepitant rales in the right lower lobe, and a protuberant abdomen. No abdominal masses could be palpated. On neurological examination she appeared restless, confused, and her ability to concentrate was poor. The motor examination revealed markedly weak iliopsoas muscles and lower leg muscles, and normal strength in the arms. All of the deep tendon reflexes were markedly hyperactive, and ankle clonus was present. The superficial abdominal reflex was absent, but the anal reflex was present. Hoffman's sign and extensor plantar responses were found bilaterally. The cranial nerves were intact. The sensory examination revealed absent vibratory sensation from the patella down bilaterally, normal vibratory sense in the hands, blunted position sense bilaterally, and normal pinprick sensation. The patient had a shuffling gait.

Laboratory test results included a hemoglobin of 13.9 gm%, hematocrit 46%, red blood cell count 4.34 million/mm³, mean corpuscular volume 102 cu μ, mean corpuscular hemoglobin concentration 30.4%, white blood cell count 7850/mm³ with 79% polymorphonuclear leukocytes, 11% lymphocytes, 5% monocytes, and 5% eosinophils. Platelets appeared normal in number on peripheral film. The serum

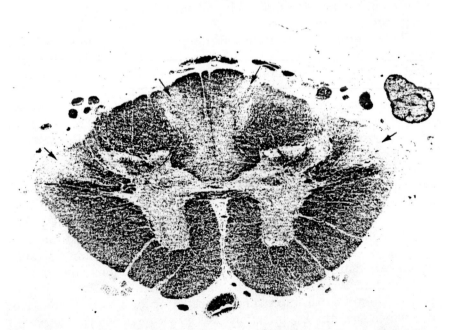

Figure 93. Section of thoracic spinal cord of a patient with subacute combined degeneration, stained with Luxol-fast blue. Areas of degeneration can be seen in the posterior and lateral column (arrows), and there is loss of both myelin and axons in these areas. (Slide courtesy of S. B. Hicks, M.D.).

B_{12} level was 153 pg/ml. A Schilling test without intrinsic factor showed 0.127% excretion of radioactivity, and there was no demonstrable free acid after histamine stimulation. Radiographic studies demonstrated a hiatus hernia of the stomach, and extensive osteoblastic lesions in the pelvis, skull, and spine.

The patient was found to be hypotensive with blood pressure of 80/50 on the third hospital day, and shortly thereafter developed fever to 102°F. Despite pressor drugs and antibiotics, she expired. At necropsy, she was found to have poorly differentiated scirrhous adenocarcinoma of the stomach with multiple metastases, and subacute combined degeneration of the spinal cord (Fig. 93).

TREATMENT

Although patients with subacute combined degeneration of the spinal cord have been treated with both liver extract and vitamin B_{12}, the response to therapy is often inconstant and unpredictable. For example, Davison[113] noted that of seven cases of subacute combined degeneration treated with liver therapy, improvement was noted in only two patients. Histopathological examination in these patients showed progressive gliosis. These changes were not seen in untreated patients with subacute combined degeneration. Myelin sheaths and axis cylinders were not influenced by liver therapy. Goldhamer et al.[166] noted that after liver therapy for pernicious anemia, symptomatic neurological improvement was noted in less than 50% of cases, and improvement of signs was seen in only 2% of cases. However, the ocular manifestations described by Cohen[93] were said to remit after therapy for pernicious anemia.

The adverse effect of folic acid upon the development and progression of subacute combined degeneration of the cord has also been noted by various investigators. Spies et al.[379] described the use of liver extract, folic acid, and thymine in pernicious anemia and subacute combined degeneration. They observed that folic acid and thymine could not prevent the development of the neurological disorder, nor relieve it once it had developed. Heinle and Welch[197] determined that folic acid could not prevent neurological relapse in some patients with pernicious anemia. In certain patients with pernicious anemia treated with folic acid, they found that the neurological manifestations were explosive in onset.

A therapeutic program for the neurological manifestations of pernicious anemia developed at the Simpson Memorial Institute and found to be effective consists of 100 micrograms of vitamin B_{12} given parenterally daily for seven days, followed by injections three times a week for four weeks. Vitamin B_{12} is then given once weekly until maximal neurological improvement occurs or for a total of one year, after which vitamin B_{12} injections are given once every two weeks indefinitely. As noted in Chapter 2, patients who demonstrate the neurological consequences of vitamin B_{12} deficiency require more intensive therapy with vitamin B_{12} than those demonstrating only hematological abnormalities.

CHAPTER 4

JUVENILE PERNICIOUS ANEMIA

Pernicious anemia in childhood is a very rare disorder. It is believed to be inherited as a homozygous recessive gene[286] and to have a male predominance.[261] It occurs in families that have a high incidence of consanguinity. This disorder usually becomes clinically evident between the ages of six and eight months. Pallor, diarrhea, anorexia, nausea, vomiting, "failure to thrive," irritability, and glossitis are among the early presenting symptoms and findings.

Achlorhydria is usually not found as consistently as it is in the adult form of pernicious anemia.[203,236,261,341] In most patients considered to have typical juvenile pernicious anemia, free acid is found in the gastric juice, and pepsin secretion is normal.[261,286] In most instances the stomach is histologically normal.[261,286]

Antibodies to intrinsic factor and to parietal cells such as those in the adult form of pernicious anemia have not been detected in juvenile pernicious anemia.[286] The primary defect in juvenile pernicious anemia is believed to be a congenital absence of intrinsic factor.[203]

Early accounts that were thought to represent childhood pernicious anemia are difficult to evaluate since essential diagnostic tests such as bone marrow aspirates and vitamin B_{12} assays were either unavailable or not performed at the time.[6,125] Cases that were more consistent with the contemporary definition of juvenile pernicious anemia and had more extensive documentation for this diagnosis appeared in the 1940s,[11,114,236,327,330] and subsequent studies more fully characterized this disorder.[38,261,286,341]

Over the years at the Simpson Memorial Institute and the University of Michigan Medical Center, two patients have been diagnosed as having juvenile pernicious anemia. The following are their case histories.

123

Case I*

This Caucasian male was born full term in 1935 after a normal spontaneous delivery. His development and appearance were normal until the age of six months when his parents noted that he was pale and irritable. Although his weight gain was normal, he vomited frequently after meals. Laboratory tests taken in 1936 when he was 1 year old revealed a hemoglobin that was 30% of normal, red blood cell count 990,000/mm^3, white blood cell count 10,000/mm^3 with 44% polymorphonuclear leukocytes, 54% lymphocytes, and 2% monocytes. He was given 12 blood transfusions elsewhere, his parents were advised that his prognosis was grave, and he was referred to the Simpson Memorial Institute for evaluation. At the time of admission he was a pale 1-year-old child in no distress. The physical examination was within normal limits.

Laboratory test results included a hemoglobin that was 55% of normal, red blood cell count 2.9 million/mm^3, and white blood cell count 9600/mm^3. Gastric lavage demonstrated no free hydrochloric acid in the gastric contents both before and after histamine stimulation. A diagnosis of "hypoplastic anemia" was made at the time, and the patient was treated with ferrous ammonium citrate.

At the age of 18 months the patient's private physician began administering injections of aqueous liver extract to him, and the anemia promptly remitted. However, injections of liver extract were given on an irregular basis, and exacerbations of the anemia occurred if the injections were omitted. In 1948, at age 12, the patient was again hospitalized at the University of Michigan Medical Center for "recurrent anemia." A bone marrow aspirate obtained several weeks after the injection of liver extract was interpreted as "normal," but the patient was suspected of having "some type of pernicious anemia."

In 1956, at age 20, the patient requested admission to the University of Michigan Medical Center so that a more firm diagnosis could be obtained prior to entry into military service. At that time, he noted that symptoms of pallor, fatigue, lightheadedness, headache, and palpitations occurred when he did not receive frequent injections of liver extract. On admission, his physical examination was within normal limits. Pertinent laboratory data included a Schilling test that demonstrated 0.3% excretion of radioactivity without intrinsic factor, and 14.8% excretion of radioactivity when vitamin B$_{12}$ was given along with pooled normal gastric juice as a source of intrinsic factor. The diagnosis of juvenile pernicious anemia was made, and the patient has subsequently maintained normal hematological values on monthly injections of vitamin B$_{12}$.

Case II**

This 4-year-old Caucasian male child was well until age 16 months when he was found to have anorexia, pallor, increased irritability, periorbital edema, and dark urine. Laboratory test results elsewhere included a hemoglobin of 4.3 gm%, hematocrit 14%, red blood cell count 1.1 million/mm^3, mean corpuscular volume 127 cubic microns, mean corpuscular hemoglobin concentration 31.3%, and reticulocyte count of 2.5%. The white blood cell count was 13,000/mm^3 with a normal differential, and the platelet count was 48,000/mm^3. The serum iron was 123 μg% and the

---

*Dr. Ronald C. Bishop made the diagnosis of juvenile pernicious anemia in this patient.

**Drs. Ruth M. Heyn and Elizabeth M. Kurczynski made the diagnosis of juvenile pernicious anemia in this patient.

total iron binding capacity was 252 μg%. A bone marrow aspirate interpreted elsewhere showed megaloblastic erythropoiesis. The patient was given a blood transfusion and sent to the University of Michigan Medical Center for evaluation. None of the patient's siblings were known to have anemia, although his mother had a "chronic anemia" of undetermined etiology.

On admission at the University of Michigan Medical Center, his physical examination was within normal limits. Laboratory test results included a hemoglobin of 9.0 gm%, hematocrit 27%, red blood cell count 2.86 million/mm^3, mean corpuscular volume 95 cubic microns, mean corpuscular hemoglobin concentration 33.3%, reticulocyte count 2.2%, white blood cell count 9400/mm^3 with a normal differential, and platelet count of 240,000/mm^3. Gastric analysis showed fasting gastric acid of 0.072 mEq acid, and after Histalog stimulation there was 0.986 mEq acid. The serum vitamin B_{12} was 15 pg/ml. A Schilling test showed 0.888% radioactivity in the urine when vitamin B_{12} alone was given, and following the Schilling test the reticulocytes rose to 25%. The patient was placed on monthly injections of vitamin B_{12} and is hematologically normal at present.

CHAPTER 5

PATHOPHYSIOLOGICAL ASPECTS OF PERNICIOUS ANEMIA

MORPHOLOGICAL ABNORMALITIES IN PERNICIOUS ANEMIA

As mentioned previously, various investigators beginning with Pepper in 1875[324] and Cohnheim in 1876[95] described the appearance of the bone marrow in pernicious anemia, insofar as they were able according to the limitations of both staining and microscopy at the time.

Following Ehrlich's identification of the megaloblast in pernicious anemia, various other authors described morphological abnormalities in cells other than erythroid precursors. In 1902, Warthin[414] described the pathology of pernicious anemia with special reference to changes occurring in the "haemolymph nodes." Warthin noted that there was prominent erythrophagocytosis in these nodes and speculated that this process might contribute to the anemia of pernicious anemia. Peabody and Broun[320] in 1925 found erythrophagocytosis in the bone marrow of patients with pernicious anemia and noted that both Cohnheim[95] and Osler and Gardner[315] had observed similar erythrophagocytosis previously. Peabody and Broun[320] stated that the intramedullary erythrophagocytosis might contribute to the pathogenesis of the anemia of pernicious anemia. Goodman et al.[171] studied bone marrow histiocytes in pernicious anemia ultrastructurally and found impressive phagocytosis of erythroid precursors in various stages of maturation and degeneration.

A number of authors have described abnormalities of megakaryocytes in pernicious anemia. Gáspár[159] in 1926 observed that in pernicious anemia there were decreased numbers of megakaryocytes. Many of them showed degenerative changes including a loss of fine

nuclear chromatin with an increase in the intensity of nuclear staining. The megakaryocytes became agranular and still later stained
homogeneously. Finally the nuclei became spherical and then
seemed to disappear. The cytoplasmic granules stained less intensely
and gradually lost their normal tinctorial properties.

In 1928, Fontana[150] noted that in pernicious anemia megakaryocytes were rare and even absent at times. Tempka and Braun[397] believed that naked megakaryocyte nuclei without cytoplasm were the
result of degenerative changes occurring in these cells. Jones[230,231]
observed that the megakaryocytes in pernicious anemia had coarse
polymorphous nuclei and intensely basophilic cytoplasm devoid of
azurophilic granules. These megakaryocytes had streaks of hyalo-
plasm and irregular areas of spongioplasm. Epstein[139] described five
cases of pernicious anemia in which there were increased numbers of
polykaryocytes (multinucleate megakaryocytes) and increased numbers of mononuclear megakaryocytes. These abnormalities were reversed after appropriate therapy.

Attention has also been focused on abnormalities of granulocytic
precursors in pernicious anemia.[18,224,230,397] Arneth[18] was the first to
describe abnormalities of polymorphonuclear leukocytes in pernicious anemia and noted that these cells both were larger and showed
greater nuclear hypersegmentation than in other disorders. Cooke[97]
later described the same cell as the "macropolycyte." Jones[230] more
fully defined the morphological characteristics and origin of this cell
and suggested that the leukocytic abnormalities were part of a pan-
myelopathy in which three different cell lines were affected. Tempka
and Braun[397] were among the first to describe gigantism of the
metamyelocyte stage of leukocyte maturation in pernicious anemia.
Although these leukocyte abnormalities are commonly sought as
characteristic morphological findings of nutritional megaloblastic
anemia, to date the factors responsible for their pathogenesis are unknown.

Beginning with Ehrlich,[129] morphological abnormalities of erythrocytes and erythroid precursors in pernicious anemia have been described in detail. The observations of Quincke,[338-340] Eichhorst,[134,135]
Laache,[257] and Cabot[64,66] have been mentioned previously (Chapter 1).
Dameshek and Valentine[111] described the primitive-appearing erythroid precursors in pernicious anemia as *erythrogones*, which they
also called *promegaloblasts*. The identity of this erythrogone and its
distinction from a proerythroblast is difficult to ascertain, but
Dameshek and Valentine believed that the erythrogone shared nuclear characteristics with primitive cells such as hemohistioblasts and
reticulum cells in addition to being larger in size than a proerythroblast. Jones,[231-233] Downey,[122] and Dacie and White[110] also described
the characteristic features of megaloblastic erythropoiesis.

Ackerman and Bellios[3] studied megaloblasts under phase contrast and found that in these cells there was an increased amount of "nucleolar associated chromatin." The significance of this observation is unclear. Fudenberg and Estren[157] described the "intermediate megaloblast" as a modified type of megaloblast, occurring primarily when iron deficiency was present concomitantly with a nutritional deficiency.

Erythroblastic gigantism has been reported in pernicious anemia by Schleicher,[365] Schwarz,[369] and Berman.[41] These authors believed that the giant erythroid forms arose as a result of abnormal suppression of cytokinesis. It has been suggested that this cytokinetic suppression may be related to defective acetylation and methylation of histones in untreated pernicious anemia erythroid precursors (Chapter 10).

CYTOCHEMICAL ABNORMALITIES IN PERNICIOUS ANEMIA

Cabot's descriptions in 1898[64] and Ehrlich's and Lazarus' observation in 1905[133] that the nucleus of the megaloblast had a decreased affinity for nuclear stains may be among the earliest observations of the unique staining properties of megaloblastic nuclear chromatin. However, there have been relatively few cytochemical studies of hematopoietic cells in pernicious anemia.

Cytochemical abnormalities of RNA in pernicious anemia megaloblasts were studied by Horrigan et al.[216] They injected vitamin B_{12} into the bone marrow of patients with untreated pernicious anemia

---

Plate 2. Rows 1 and 2: Abnormalities of nucleic acids and histones in pernicious anemia megaloblasts. *Row 1, left:* Large proerythroblasts and early intermediate megaloblasts stained with methyl green-pyronin. The intensely pyroninophilic cytoplasm (red) indicates increased content of RNA. The RNA appears in large aggregates. *Row 1, right:* Feulgen-stained megaloblasts showing magenta-colored delicate-appearing strands of DNA and few aggregates of DNA. *Row 2, left:* Ammoniacal silver-stained proerythroblast or early intermediate megaloblast showing predominantly lysine-rich histone (yellow-staining material) in the nucleus. *Row 2, right:* Alkaline-fast green-stained megaloblasts illustrating a delicate network of green-staining histone threads and few aggregates of histones.

Plate 2. Rows 3 and 4: Abnormalities of cytoplasmic constituents in pernicious anemia megaloblasts. *Row 3, left:* Alizarine red S-stained megaloblasts, showing pink staining of the cytoplasm. This pink staining may be due in large part to the increased content of methylmalonyl CoA in these cells and may therefore be cytochemical evidence of a metabolic block in the coenzyme B_{12}-dependent methylmalonyl CoA mutase enzyme. *Row 3, right:* Strong nonspecific esterase activity (red orange) in the cytoplasm of pernicious anemia megaloblasts. *Row 4, left:* PAS stain demonstrating glycogen (red orange) in the cytoplasm of megaloblasts and proerythroblasts. Both diffuse and punctate PAS positivity are observed. *Row 4, right:* Phosphorylase (amylophosphorylase) activity in proerythroblasts and early intermediate megaloblasts in pernicious anemia. The violet brown cytoplasmic granules represent phosphorylase activity. Increased amounts of phosphorylase in pernicious anemia may be among the factors contributing to the pathogenesis of the deposits of glycogen detectable as PAS positive material in these cells.

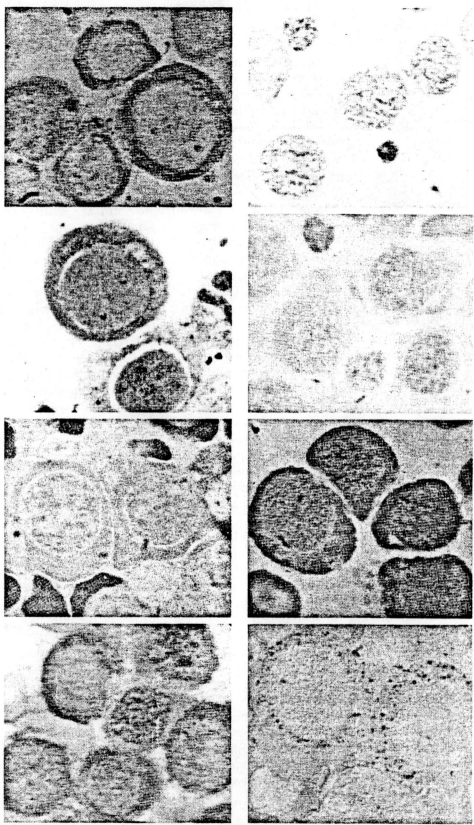

See legend on the opposite page.

129

and then repeated a marrow aspiration after 48 hours from the same site and from the opposite iliac crest. These authors found that in untreated megaloblasts, cytoplasmic RNA visualized with the pyronin stain appeared block-like and granular (Plate 2). After treatment with vitamin B_{12}, the RNA appeared diffuse and homogeneous.

Cytochemically, DNA may be demonstrated with the use of the Feulgen reagent. Staining of pernicious anemia erythroid precursors with this reagent demonstrates a network of thin-appearing magenta colored strands with few aggregates of DNA at points of junction of the strands (Plate 2 and Fig. 107). These strands of DNA are more attenuated-appearing, and the aggregates of chromatin are smaller than in normoblasts at a comparable stage of maturation.

The alkaline-fast green stain has been used to demonstrate histone in pernicious anemia megaloblasts.[239] This stain reveals a network of delicate-appearing histone strands and few aggregates of histones as illustrated in Plate 2 and Figure 113.

In investigating the type of histones in pernicious anemia megaloblasts and in erythroid precursors in other types of anemia, the ammoniacal silver stain was used to distinguish between lysine-rich and arginine-rich histones on the basis of color differences. One study[239] determined that proerythroblasts and early intermediate megaloblasts in pernicious anemia were unique in that they contained abundant lysine-rich histone. This type of histone imparted a yellow color to the nucleus (Plate 2). Brown speckled areas representing arginine-rich histone were observed rarely. These cytochemical observations served as the initial stimulus for other biochemical studies involving histone biosynthesis in pernicious anemia (see Chapter 10).

A recent study[243] investigated cytoplasmic components of megaloblasts in pernicious anemia using the anthraquinone dye alizarine red S. Formalin-fixation of films of marrow followed by staining with a solution of alizarine red S produced a unique pink colored staining of the cytoplasm of megaloblasts in untreated pernicious anemia (Plate 2). This pink colored cytoplasmic staining was not observed either in folate deficiency or in a variety of other types of anemias including the DiGuglielmo syndrome. After treatment of the pernicious anemia with vitamin B_{12}, the cytoplasm of the macronormoblasts appeared yellow, suggesting that the substance responsible for the pink color in the untreated megaloblasts decreased in amount or disappeared after treatment with vitamin B_{12}.

With the use of test tube experiments involving a wide variety of potential substrates that might be found in pernicious anemia megaloblasts as well as other types of erythroid precursors, it was found that a deep rose pink color occurred with several metabolic intermediates of the pentose-phosphate shunt pathway, as well as the citric acid cycle and the Embden-Meyerhof pathway. A particular and perhaps significant finding was that methylmalonyl-CoA produced a rose color. Since this compound is known to be increased in vitamin B_{12}–deficient cells due to a metabolic block in the 5'-deoxy-adenosylcobalamin-dependent enzyme methylmalonyl-CoA mutase,[373] it was postulated that the cytoplasmic pinkness of megaloblasts stained with alizarine red S may be cytochemical evidence of a metabolic block occurring in pernicious anemia. On the basis of these experiments, it was suggested that methylmalonyl-CoA was probably one of the more important of several metabolic intermediates that might be responsible for the pink cytoplasmic color.

Activity of nonspecific esterase enzyme using alpha-naphthyl acetate as the substrate has been found to be increased in the cytoplasm of pernicious anemia megaloblasts by Rosenszajn et al.[355] as illustrated in Plate 2. The significance of this increased nonspecific esterase activity in megaloblasts is uncertain, but it is believed to relate to a disturbance in the regulation of protein synthesis in pernicious anemia.[355] Similar increased nonspecific esterase activity has been found in the erythroid precursors of the DiGuglielmo syndrome.[244,355]

Periodic acid-Schiff (PAS) positive material can often be demonstrated in the cytoplasm of pernicious anemia megaloblasts (Plate 2). This PAS positivity indicating increased amounts of glycogen may appear in either a diffuse or granular pattern. Reasons why glycogen is increased in vitamin B_{12}–deficient erythroid precursors are unclear, but they may perhaps relate to abnormalities in glycogenolytic enzymes such as amylophosphorylase that would normally degrade glycogen.

Recent studies performed in collaboration with Dr. M. Hadi have suggested that one of these enzymes involved in the glycogen pathway may be abnormal in PAS-positive megaloblasts in pernicious anemia.[248] As illustrated in Plate 2, phosphorylase a (amylophosphorylase) activity was visualized as coarse granular-appearing violet brown particles in the cytoplasm of proerythroblasts and early intermediate megaloblasts in pernicious anemia. Diffuse violet to brown staining of megaloblast cytoplasm was also observed. Phosphorylase activity was detected most readily in the cytoplasm of early erythroid precursors in pernicious anemia, although occasional late intermediate megaloblasts showed evidence of activity. Increased phosphorylase activity was not found in erythroid precursors obtained from normal individuals or from patients with a wide variety of anemias in which the erythroid precursors were PAS-negative. However, increased phosphorylase activity was found in a pattern similar to that seen in pernicious anemia in megaloblastoid erythroid precursors in chronic erythremic myelosis (DiGuglielmo syndrome). In these erythroid precursors and in pernicious anemia megaloblasts, the most intense phosphorylase activity was found in erythroid precursors that showed the most intense PAS staining.

Under normal circumstances, phosphorylase is believed to function primarily in the degradation of glycogen, although the reaction may also proceed in the opposite direction, i.e., toward glycogen synthesis. It is conceivable that in erythroid precursors whose metabolism is disturbed as in chronic erythremic myelosis and pernicious anemia, phosphorylase activity may be abnormally increased, as shown in Plate 2. In these metabolically abnormal cells, the synthesis rather than degradation of glycogen may be facilitated by increased phosphorylase, leading to deposits of glycogen detectable by the PAS reagent.

The Prussian blue reagent used to detect the presence of iron often demonstrates multiple coarse siderotic granules in megaloblasts in untreated pernicious anemia (Fig. 123). These ringed sideroblasts constitute cytochemical evidence of disturbed iron metabolism and ineffective erythropoiesis in pernicious anemia (Chapter 10) as well as in other types of anemia.[244] Iron metabolism has been studied cytochemically in pernicious anemia bone marrow histiocytes and a unique pattern of small iron granules 0.3 micron in diameter occurring singly or in aggregates was observed in the cytoplasm of these cells.[413] Subsequent ultrastructural studies demonstrated that this iron was present in vesicles.[171]

Various enzymes of bone marrow cells in megaloblastic anemias have been detected using cytochemical techniques.[385] In megaloblasts from patients with pernicious anemia, activities of enzymes indicated by the deposition of formazan salts were increased in the Embden-Meyerhof, pentose phosphate shunt, and Krebs cycle pathways in all megaloblasts at all stages of maturation. Specific enzymes found to be increased were lactic dehydrogenase, malic dehydrogenase, succinic dehydrogenase, alpha GPD-M, alpha GPD-S, glucose-6-phosphate dehydrogenase, and 6-phosphogluconic acid dehydrogenase. It was suggested that the marked elevation of serum LDH in pernicious anemia could be caused in part by destruction of megaloblasts containing large amounts of lactic dehydrogenase. The latter study[385] may provide a cytochemical explanation for the increased serum levels of malic dehydrogenase and 6-phosphogluconic acid dehydrogenase that occur in the serum of pernicious anemia patients.[199] Elevations in serum levels of fructolase, phosphohexose isomerase, and isocitric dehydrogenase are also found in pernicious anemia,[199] as are increased levels of muramidase.[325]

CYTOGENETIC ABNORMALITIES IN PERNICIOUS ANEMIA

Various authors have described chromosomal aberrations in patients with untreated pernicious anemia.[23,55,152,196,254,290,331] Although these abnormalities are probably nonspecific, they are believed to reflect the disorder of nucleic acid synthesis as well as mitotic divisions that occur in pernicious anemia.

Astaldi et al.[23] observed 100 metaphase plates in untreated pernicious anemia bone marrows. Of these 100 plates, 19 had 46 chromosomes, 11 had 45 chromosomes, and 50 had 44 chromosomes. The authors also observed monosomy of the fifth and twelfth pairs, absence of both chromsomes of group 20, monosomy for chromosome 15, and absence of one X and apparent absence of both X chromosomes. Acentric fragments and occasional secondary constrictions simulating dicentric chromosomes were also found. After treatment[24,25] it was found that the chromosomal abnormalities largely disappeared. However, some hypodiploid cells were seen. Powsner and Berman[331] observed that the chromosomes in pernicious anemia were approximately 30% longer than normal chromosomes.

Kiossoglou et al.[254] studied three cases of pernicious anemia before and after therapy. In untreated cases they observed chromatid gaps, giant chromosomes, aneuploidy (44 and 45 chromosomes), and monosomy involving G21 chromosomes. Similar chromosomal aberrations were found in tissues other than erythroid precursors in their study, indicating that the disturbances resulting from deficiency of vitamin B_{12} were widespread.

Menzies et al.[290] studied the cytogenetic and cytochemical abnormalities in the bone marrow in vitamin B_{12} and folate deficiency. They did not observe an increase in aneuploidy. However, they found an arrest of DNA synthesis in some cells, and in others found a prolongation of S and G_2. In addition, there were chromatid breaks showing no reunion and preference for the centromeric region. These breaks occurred at sites of secondary constriction. Increased size of centromeric constriction was seen. At the normal sites of secondary constriction, there was marked negative heteropyknosis that appeared as large gaps. Satellites of acrocentric chromosomes were found, as were thin elongated chromosomes. Bottura and Coutinho[55] found gaps or breaks of the chromatid and chromosome types and acentric fragments, but there was no obvious tendency to localization of the breaks in certain areas.

GENETICS OF PERNICIOUS ANEMIA

From the early studies of Levine and Ladd[273] in 1921, it had been appreciated that there were strong familial tendencies in pernicious anemia and that pernicious anemia seemed to occur more frequently in individuals of British or Scandinavian descent. Other anthropomorphic studies[123,189] suggested that blue eyes, low set ears, acromegaloid features, and premature graying or whitening of the hair are frequently observed in patients with pernicious anemia, but these findings are by no means invariable.

The actual genetic mechanisms in pernicious anemia are not well understood. In one report 106 relatives of 34 patients with pernicious anemia were studied.[287] Schilling tests[364] were performed on all of these patients to note any defects in vitamin B_{12} absorption. It was stated that the relatives of the pernicious anemia patients had abnormal Schilling tests more frequently than controls. Also, the number of relatives with abnormal vitamin B_{12} absorption increased with advancing chronological age. It was concluded that the predisposition to pernicious anemia was inherited as a single autosomal dominant factor. Recently, these original findings of abnormal Schilling tests in relatives of patients with pernicious anemia have been retracted by McIntyre.[288]

Whittingham et al.[430] studied genetic factors in pernicious anemia as related to gastritis. They found that the gastric lesion of pernicious anemia was determined by (1) nonspecific damaging environmental agents and (2) an inherited defect in the immunological tolerance to a specific complex of antigens, leading to an autoimmune reaction to gastric components. In the opinion of these authors, to make the transition from gastritis to pernicious anemia an interaction between the two factors had to take place. Only certain predisposed individuals underwent this transition, whereas others demonstrated only gastritis.

CELLULAR KINETIC ABNORMALITIES
IN PERNICIOUS ANEMIA

Studies of erythrocyte production and destruction in pernicious anemia have supported the concept that the anemia in pernicious anemia is characterized by ineffective erythropoiesis. In this condition, as defined by Finch et al.,[109,145] although total erythropoietic activity may be elevated, intramedullary destruction of erythrocytes occurs, and insufficient functional erythrocytes are delivered to the peripheral blood. Cytological evidence for intramedullary destruction of erythroid precursors in pernicious anemia can be found in the numerous degenerating megaloblasts (Chapter 2) and in the erythrophagocytosis of both erythrocytes and megaloblasts, as noted by various early investigators including Cohnheim,[95] Osler and Gardner,[315] and Peabody and Broun[320] (Chapter 1).

Finch et al.[145] studied erythrokinetics in pernicious anemia and found that the total erythropoietic activity was approximately three times normal. However, the delivery of viable erythrocytes to the peripheral blood was abnormal, accounting for the anemia and representing ineffective erythropoiesis. Total erythropoietic activity was reflected by turnover of heme components. The rate of destruction of erythrocytes was found to be three times normal. All of these factors were believed to contribute to the pathogenesis of the anemia of pernicious anemia. The reticulocyte count was found to be an unreliable index of blood production in patients with untreated pernicious anemia because the reticulum of the reticulocyte was often lost prior to entry of the young erythrocyte into the circulation. After therapy with vitamin B_{12}, erythropoiesis increased to three or four times normal and became *effective*.

Myhre[307] observed the proliferation and destruction of nucleated erythroid precursors in pernicious anemia before and during treatment with vitamin B_{12}. A markedly increased destruction of nucleated erythroid precursors was observed in untreated pernicious anemia, supporting the postulate that intramedullary hemolysis was important in the pathogenesis of the anemia of this disorder.

In a second study the maturation time of megaloblasts, as measured by the disappearance rate of basophilic and polychromatophilic erythroblasts and by radioactive iron uptake, was found to be moderately prolonged in pernicious anemia.[308] There was a failure in accumulation of orthochromatic erythroblasts, and a relatively low incorporation of ^{59}Fe into hemoglobin during incubation of the pernicious anemia erythroid precursors. It was postulated that the destruction of erythroblasts occurred mainly at the late polychromatophilic or orthochromatic stages of development. These parameters normalized after two or more days of treatment with vitamin B_{12}.

Nathan and Gardner[309] studied erythroid cell maturation and hemoglobin synthesis in megaloblastic anemia. Using ^{14}C glycine and ^{59}Fe to measure hemoglobin and globin synthesis and erythrocyte maturation time, they found, as did Myhre[308] and Astaldi,[22] that the maturation time of the megaloblast was prolonged. This prolongation was more marked at the early stages of maturation and became more normal as the erythroid precursor matured. Hemoglobin and globin syntheses were synchronous, and vitamin B_{12} was found to shorten the maturation time.

Rondanelli et al.[350] reported the differences in the proliferative activity between normoblasts and pernicious anemia megaloblasts. It was observed that the duration of mitosis in megaloblasts was shorter than in normoblasts, confirming the tissue culture studies of Astaldi.[22] This shortening of the duration of mitosis was found in every stage of erythroid maturation. The proliferative activity in pernicious anemia was markedly increased compared to normal, since the generation time was inversely proportional to the frequency by which new mitoses were entered into a cell population.

Messner et al.[291] described the kinetics of erythropoietic cell proliferation in pernicious anemia. Using tritiated thymidine studies *in vivo*, the initial tritiated thymidine labeling index of the more mature erythroid precursor compartment was lower in pernicious anemia patients than in normal persons. The lower limit of average DNA synthesis time in pernicious anemia was 13 hours and the upper limit of generation time was 21 hours. There was a lower increment of labeling per unit time in the compartments E3 to E5 in megaloblasts when compared to normoblasts.

Messner et al.[291] interpreted their results as indicating that there were two erythroblast populations in pernicious anemia, probably identical morphologically. One population progressed normally and was "in cycle." The other population was believed to be "out of cycle," and it was this particular population that underwent a high death rate of cells and was believed to contribute significantly to the pathogenesis of the anemia of pernicious anemia.

Wickramasinghe et al.[431,432] found disturbances of the proliferation of erythroid cells in pernicious anemia and found a decreased S/G_2 ratio in the early polychromatophilic megaloblasts caused by a relative increase in the number of cells in G_2. There was an increased proportion of unlabeled cells with DNA contents that were between the 2c and 4c modes. Several cells did not demonstrate DNA synthesis. These changes were less pronounced in the promegaloblasts and basophilic megaloblasts than in the dividing polychromatophilic megaloblasts. The authors postulated that the failure of DNA synthesis in the G_2 phase led to death of these cells and accounted in part for the ineffective erythropoiesis in pernicious anemia.

Yoshida et al.[444] examined the proliferation of megaloblasts in pernicious anemia as measured by their nucleic acid metabolism. By microspectrophotometric estimates, DNA contents were increased in cells with DNA values around the 4c value. Autoradiographic experiments using tritiated thymidine demonstrated a decreased ability of megaloblasts to synthesize DNA. It was postulated that there was impaired DNA synthesis with occasional arrests of synthesis as well as prolongation of the S period with or without the prolongation of G_2. There was active incorporation of tritiated uridine and tritiated leucine, indicating that RNA and protein synthesis were probably active and relatively unaffected compared to the abnormalities in DNA synthesis. All of the DNA synthesis abnormalities were corrected by vitamin B_{12}.

In a separate study, Wickramasinghe et al.[433] studied the arrest of cell proliferation and protein synthesis in megaloblasts of pernicious anemia. A proportion of megaloblasts were found in G_2, and the cells that were apparently arrested after the period of DNA synthesis showed little or no evidence of protein synthesis. The authors interpreted their findings as indicating that these particular cells were arrested in the cell cycle and destined for an intramedullary cell death. A marked depression of protein synthesis was seen in some G_1 cells. The arrest of cell proliferation in pernicious anemia occurred at all stages of interphases. It was also concluded that the reticulocyte response in treated pernicious anemia was largely the result of the maturation of a new generation of erythroid cells or of the most immature basophilic erythroblasts that were least affected insofar as the cell cycle and the arrest in protein synthesis were seen. Intramedullary destruction occurred predominantly in the polychromatophilic megaloblast stages of maturation.

Cooper and Wickramasinghe[102] investigated the quantitative cytochemistry of pernicious anemia megaloblasts in their investigations of the erythrokinetic abnormalities in pernicious anemia. An increased number of cells were noted in G_2, but some cells were not in a phase of DNA synthesis. These cells did not incorporate tritiated thymidine and were called U cells. The defects were maximal in the early polychromatophilic megaloblast stage, as had been determined in earlier studies[431-433] and noted by Myhre.[307,308] The authors suggested that the U cells represented cells that were arrested in G_2 and might account in large part for the ineffective erythropoiesis seen in pernicious anemia.

Although erythrokinetic abnormalities have been studied extensively in pernicious anemia, there have also been several reports indicating that the kinetics of granulocytes and platelets may be disturbed in this disorder. In addition to ineffective erythropoiesis occurring in pernicious anemia, various authors have proposed that an ineffective granulopoiesis also occurs.[275,325,434] Liu and Sullivan[275] administered *Pseudomonas* polysaccharide to patients with pernicious anemia and to normal patients in an effort to study granulocyte reserve in the bone marrow. In patients with pernicious anemia, the polymorphonuclear leukocytes showed a minimal response to the endotoxin compared to the response seen in normal individuals. Perillie et al.[325] extended these observations and found that muramidase (lysozyme) was increased in the serum of patients with untreated pernicious anemia. They postulated that since most of the serum muramidase was derived from degraded granulocytes, the leukopenia and granulocytopenia in pernicious anemia probably resulted from increased granulocyte turnover and death of giant metamyelocytes in the bone marrow.

Recently, Wickramasinghe and Pratt[434] helped to clarify some of the mechanisms responsible for this ineffective granulopoiesis. In an autoradiographic and spectroscopic study of nucleic acid metabolism in pernicious anemia granulocyte precursors, they found that pernicious anemia myelocytes had a prolonged S period. In 15% to 30% of the giant metamyelocytes, there was a gross slowing of DNA synthesis. A high proportion of these giant metamyelocytes were found to be in G_2, probably representing a premitotic arrest. The authors stated that because of the bizarre nuclear morphology of the giant metamyelocytes, weak labeling with tritiated thymidine, and a "pile up" in G_2, the giant metamyelocyte was probably a degenerating cell that underwent intramedullary cell death.[275,434] An example of phagocytosis of these giant metamyelocytes by histiocytic cells in the bone marrow of a patient with pernicious anemia is illustrated in Figure 94.

Wickramasinghe's and Pratt's study[434] also indicated that the giant

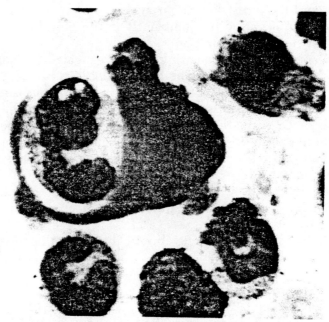

Figure 94.   Phagocytosis of giant aberrant-appearing metamyelocyte by large phago-
cyte in the bone marrow of a patient with severe pernicious anemia. This phagocytosis
may constitute cytological evidence for the ineffective granulopoiesis and increased
serum levels of muramidase (lysozyme) and lactic dehydrogenase seen in severe pernicious anemia.

metamyelocytes in pernicious anemia were often hyperdiploid,
whereas the circulating hypersegmented polymorphonuclear leukocyte in pernicious anemia had only a diploid DNA content. They
concluded that the hypersegmented polymorphonuclear leukocyte
was not derived from the maturation of the giant metamyelocytes
without cellular division but arose from maturation of diploid metamyelocytes having normal morphology.

   In terms of platelets, Harker and Finch[190] studied thrombokinetics in pernicious anemia as well as other hematopoietic disorders. It
was found that the megakaryocyte mass was increased in pernicious
anemia but that the production of platelets as measured by platelet
turnover was decreased. This discrepancy between total production
(megakaryocyte mass) and platelet production (platelet turnover) was
believed to indicate "ineffective thrombopoiesis." The finding of degenerating megakaryocytes in untreated pernicious anemia marrows[150,159,230,231,397] suggests the possibility that intramedullary destruction of megakaryocytes may also contribute to the development of
thrombocytopenia in this disorder. Examples of these degenerating
megakaryocytes in pernicious anemia bone marrows are illustrated in
Figure 95.

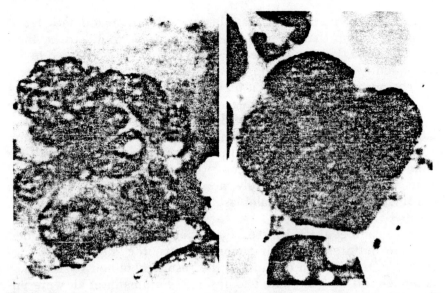

Figure 95. Degenerating megakaryocytes from the bone marrow of a patient with severe pernicious anemia. *Left:* the nucleus has become fragmented and the nuclear chromatin unusually coarse. There are tenuous-appearing connections between nuclear lobes, and the nucleus appears to be disintegrating. *Right:* condensations of nuclear chromatin and loss of cytoplasm are seen.

TISSUE CULTURE STUDIES IN PERNICIOUS ANEMIA

A number of tissue culture studies involving marrow cells from patients with pernicious anemia have been performed. Many of these studies have provided useful information regarding parameters of protein synthesis and cellular maturation in the pernicious anemia erythroid precursors.

Lajtha[258] described an inhibiting factor in pernicious anemia serum, whereby a "factor" in untreated pernicious anemia serum inhibited the "ripening" (conversion) of megaloblasts to normoblasts in tissue cultures in which normal serum was used. This same factor was believed to convert normoblasts to megaloblasts in cultures. The factor was found to be thermostable and was recovered from the cerebrospinal fluid of patients with relapsed pernicious anemia. Folic acid and liver extract were said to overcome the inhibitory influence of the factor, but vitamin B_{12} did not. Thompson[399] confirmed Lajtha's experiments by demonstrating an "agent" in pernicious anemia plasma that was capable of inhibiting the maturation of megaloblasts into normoblasts in tissue cultures containing normal serum. He observed that this agent could "annul" the maturing effect of normal plasma.

Callender and Lajtha[68] found that incubation of normal gastric juice with vitamin B_{12} produced a thermolabile factor that ripened megaloblasts in tissue cultures. If gastric juice and vitamin B_{12} were

used separately, no ripening was observed. The hematopoietic factor .
in normal serum that ripened megaloblasts was found to be thermolabile. It has been suggested that this factor may be related to the
subsequently isolated vitamin B_{12} transport proteins.[184]

Thompson[400] reported that only folic acid had a direct maturing
effect on pernicious anemia megaloblasts in tissue culture. Vitamin
B_{12}, thymidine, and liver extract did not show this maturing effect.
Lajtha[259] demonstrated the reversibility between normoblastic and
megaloblastic cells in tissue cultures of human bone marrow. He
found that megaloblasts could convert to normoblasts when normal
serum was used and, conversely, normoblasts could convert to cells
indistinguishable from megaloblasts when pernicious anemia serum
was used.

Feinmann et al.[143] observed that when normal serum was added
to tissue cultures containing megaloblasts, the megaloblasts decreased in number. In contrast to the results obtained by Lajtha,[258]
Callender and Lajtha,[68] and Thompson,[399] Feinmann et al. were unable to demonstrate an "inhibitory factor."

Astaldi[22] found that megaloblasts incubated in tissue cultures containing pernicious anemia serum showed a delayed maturation. Addition of nicotinamide or liver extract to the culture led to normalization
of maturation. With the addition of nicotinamide, the megaloblastosis
persisted although maturation appeared to progress normally. Addition of normal serum to pernicious anemia cells led to normoblastic
transformation, as others[68,258,259] had observed previously. Addition of
vitamin B_{12} to cultures containing pernicious anemia serum and
megaloblasts did not lead to conversion. Astaldi's findings support the
earlier studies of Lajtha, Callender and Lajtha, and Thompson who
found that pernicious anemia serum contained an inhibitory factor
that prevented the conversion of megaloblasts to normoblasts. To
date, the nature of this inhibitory factor has not been fully defined.

Astaldi[22] also reported that megaloblasts proliferated more actively in tissue cultures than normoblasts at both basophilic and polychromatophilic states of maturation. This proliferation was twice as
great as normoblastic maturation in the basophilic stage, and four
times greater than normoblastic maturation in the polychromatophilic
stage. Astaldi also noted that the duration of mitosis was shorter in
pernicious anemia than in normal erythroid precursors.

Falabella et al.[140] studied the conversion of megaloblasts into
normoblasts in tissue culture after adding various forms of vitamin B_{12},
including coenzyme B_{12} (5'-deoxyadenosylcobalamin), methylcobalamin, and cyanocobalamin. They observed that megaloblasts
converted most readily to normoblasts in tissue culture when coenzyme B_{12} was added and postulated that coenzyme B_{12} had a direct
effect on megaloblasts.

BILE PIGMENT METABOLISM IN PERNICIOUS ANEMIA

There have been several studies of bile pigment metabolism in pernicious anemia. The most recent of these studies have suggested that intramedullary destruction of erythrocytes accounts in large part for the abnormalities of biliary pigment found in pernicious anemia.

Clinically, hyperbilirubinemia with frank icterus can be observed in cases of severe pernicious anemia, and the decline in bile pigments in the blood was one of the parameters that Minot and Murphy[298] originally used to assess the efficacy of liver therapy in pernicious anemia. As mentioned earlier, Whipple[425,428] originally believed that the increased stercobilin production in pernicious anemia resulted from increased production of cells rather than increased destruction.

London and West[277] subsequently reported that in untreated pernicious anemia, a large part of the bile pigment was derived from one or more sources other than the hemoglobin of the mature, circulating erythrocytes. These investigators used ^{15}N labeled glycine and found that the mean erythrocyte survival in pernicious anemia was 85 days, the rate of production of erythrocyte hemoglobin was 80% of normal, and the rate of production of circulating erythrocytes was 50% of normal. There was strikingly high ^{15}N stercobilin excretion in the stool from the fifth to the twelfth days of the study. They also found that the increased coproporphyrin I excretion returned to normal after treatment with liver extract. London and West's findings may be interpreted as demonstrating the intramedullary destruction of erythrocytes and probably erythroid precursors in pernicious anemia.

NUCLEIC ACID ABNORMALITIES IN PERNICIOUS ANEMIA

Various studies have demonstrated that there is defective biosynthesis of DNA in untreated pernicious anemia megaloblasts and that this abnormality can be corrected with the administration of vitamin B_{12}. Several initial studies were concerned with the hematological effects of DNA precursors, such as thymine, in pernicious anemia. Spies et al.[380] reported that thymine could induce a remission in a patient with untreated pernicious anemia. In a series of investigations relating to nucleic acid abnormalities in pernicious anemia, Vilter et al.[410] determined that megaloblasts were deficient in DNA and especially in thymine. They observed that both uracil and thymine led to a remission in pernicious anemia and that partial responses were obtained with methionine and choline. They postulated that folic acid acted as a coenzyme concerned with the formation of DNA from precursors such as uracil, purines, and thymine. Vitamin B_{12} was then believed to activate the formation of nucleosides (thymidine) from the purines and pyrimidines to form nucleic acids.

Vilter et al.[410] also studied the relationships between vitamin B_{12}, folic acid, and various nucleoside intermediates. They found that patients with pernicious anemia maintained on folic acid for two to three years suffered hematological relapses that remitted on liver extract, folate, or thymine. They postulated that folic acid was essential to the formation of thymine and other pyrimidines and purines. Manifestations of spinal cord lesions appeared in all patients with pernicious anemia who received continuing folate therapy. Uracil led to a remission of the relapsed pernicious anemia.

White et al.[429] observed that DNA-phosphorus was increased in pernicious anemia erythroid cells, and RNA-phosphorus was also above normal but decreased toward normal with increasing cellular maturity during therapy for the pernicious anemia. Glazer et al.[165] studied the effect of vitamin B_{12} and folic acid on the nucleic acid composition of the bone marrow of patients with megaloblastic anemias. They found that of 11 pernicious anemia marrows from which nucleoproteins had been extracted, the RNA/DNA and uracil/thymine ratios were higher than normal. The relative amounts of thymine were lower than normal. After treatment the RNA/DNA and uracil/thymine ratios fell, and thymine increased to normal.

Spray and Witts[381] investigated the role of thymidine in megaloblastic anemias. They found that intramuscular thymidine given in doses of 250 milligrams daily for ten days produced a slight hematopoietic response in a patient with relapsed pernicious anemia. In several other patients, however, even higher doses of thymidine did not produce an effect.

Lajtha and Kumatori[260] studied nucleic acid metabolism in pernicious anemia *in vitro*. Using autoradiographic techniques, they found that DNA synthesis was slightly increased in megaloblasts but not in myelocytes. The synthesis of RNA was greatly increased in myelocytes and even more so in megaloblasts. Thomas and Lochte[398] found that vitamin B_{12} affected DNA synthesis but not oxygen consumption or heme synthesis. They found that vitamin B_{12} had a direct although unexplained effect on DNA synthesis and that pernicious anemia serum did not appear to inhibit DNA synthesis in megaloblasts exposed to vitamin B_{12}. In contrast to the results obtained by others[292] Lessner and Friedkin[272] demonstrated that uridine and thymidine uptakes were normal in megaloblastic marrow. No impairment of uridine methylation or thymidine incorporation was observed after addition of vitamin B_{12} or folate.

In a series of studies beginning in 1961, Beck[30-36] postulated that a lack of vitamin B_{12} led to what he called *unbalanced growth* in certain bacteria having an absolute requirement for vitamin B_{12}. Lack of vitamin B_{12} in growth media led to the formation of filamentous microorganisms. Beck suggested that there was an analogy between these structures and the pathogenesis of the delicate chromatin found in megaloblasts. Beck et al.[31] found that addition of vitamin B_{12} to previously limited cultures of *Lactobacillus leichmannii* caused an increase in DNA concentration and increase in the ratio of DNA/RNA and DNA/protein and an increased concentration of acid-soluble deoxyribosides, ribonucleotides, and unidentified compounds containing deoxyribosyl moieties in combined forms. The acid-soluble deoxyribosyl compounds were DNA precursors and vitamin B_{12} functioned primarily in their biosynthesis. If nutritional repletion with vitamin B_{12} took place after more than two hours of unbalanced growth in the deficient media, the filamentous growth in the bacteria was not fully reversed despite the extensive replacement of DNA.

Beck et al.[32] subsequently found that vitamin B_{12} or deoxyriboside starvation led to long, nonviable filaments with decreased DNA/RNA and DNA/protein ratios. Excess vitamin B_{12} or deoxyriboside increased DNA synthesis and led to unusually small viable forms with increased DNA/RNA and DNA/protein ratios. Replacement of free purines and pyrimidines with corresponding ribosides in cultures containing vitamin B_{12} led to unusually small forms with normal DNA/RNA and increased DNA/protein and RNA/protein, whereas riboside substitution had no such effect in deoxyriboside cultures. These authors concluded that vitamin B_{12} participated in the conversion of ribosyl to deoxyribosyl groups.

Reisner and Korson[342] found that DNA was not increased in megaloblasts and that with increasing maturation DNA was gradually lost from the megaloblast nuclei. In five patients with pernicious anemia, hydroxycobalamin added to cultures of bone marrow stimulated the incorporation of labeled ^{14}C adenine and cytidine into DNA bases but not into RNA bases.

A number of recent studies of the role of deoxyuridine in the synthesis of thymine DNA have shed light on possible mechanisms contributing to the pathogenesis of megaloblastic erythropoiesis. Donohue and Azzam[120] initially found that the rate of incorporation of deoxyuridine compared to thymidine increased threefold in pernicious anemia marrows after exposure to vitamin B_{12}. They concluded that vitamin B_{12} enhanced the conversion of deoxyuridine to thymidine. Subsequently, Killmann[253] demonstrated that the addition of deoxyuridine to cultures of normal marrow erythroid cells caused an 80% to 100% decrease in the uptake of tritiated thymidine, whereas the addition of deoxyuridine to cultures of pernicious anemia megaloblasts had little or no effect on tritiated thymidine uptake. Killmann stated that in vitamin B_{12} deficiency, the methylation of deoxyuridylic acid to thymidylic acid was defective. Presumably, the mechanism of the block in tritiated thymidine uptake in Killmann's studies was the increase in the thymidylate pool accompanying the addition of a large amount of deoxyuridine to the system, resulting in decreased uptake of tritiated thymidine into DNA.

Metz et al.[292] further clarified the mechanisms by which the addition of deoxyuridine to cultures of megaloblasts did not lead to the normal suppression of DNA synthesis as judged by tritiated thymidine uptake. Metz et al. showed that there was defective incorporation of deoxyuridine into thymine DNA in vitamin B_{12} and folate deficient bone marrows. The defect was corrected by vitamin B_{12} only in the vitamin B_{12} deficient marrows and completely corrected by folic acid (PGA but not methyltetrahydrofolate) in both. Methotrexate blocked the corrective effect of vitamin B_{12}.

The authors stated that in normal subjects the deoxyuridine entered the deoxyuridine → thymidine → thymine DNA pathway, so that the incorporation into DNA of labeled tritiated thymidine monophosphate derived from the added tritiated thymidine was diminished. However, in pernicious anemia there was an abnormality in the synthesis of thymine DNA from deoxyuridine. This abnormality was believed to be caused by the lack of folate intermediates, particularly 5,10-methylenetetrahydrofolate, that are necessary for the methylation of deoxyuridine monophosphate to form thymine monophosphate. A reduction in activity of the methylcobalamin-dependent N^5-methyltetrahydrofolate-homocysteine methyltransferase was thought to be a primary factor leading to reduced amounts of folate intermediates. Because of the lack of these folate intermediates, the addition of deoxyuridine to cultures of megaloblasts did not have the normal blocking effect on tritiated thymidine uptake. The reactions may be diagrammed as follows:

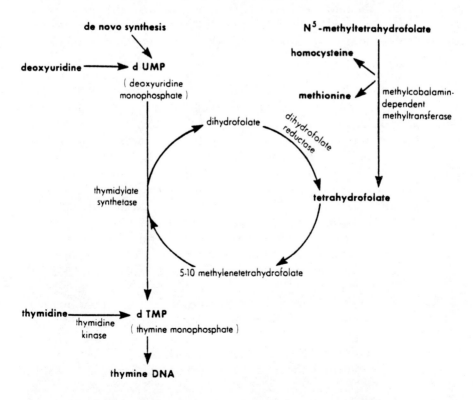

Presumably, the resulting defect in DNA synthesis leads to megaloblastosis.[292]

Metz et al. stated that these studies supported the *methyltetrahydrofolate trap* hypothesis (Chapter 10) since N^5-methyltetrahydrofolate failed to correct the defect in DNA synthesis. They also concluded that in man, riboside reduction may be independent of vitamin B_{12}. Waxman et al.[415] found that in vitamin B_{12}–deficient bone marrow cells there was inadequate DNA synthesis due to a block in tetrahydrofolic acid regeneration from N^5-methyltetrahydrofolate via homocysteine methylation.

Other enzymes involved in the biosynthesis of DNA have also been found to be abnormal in pernicious anemia. Bock et al.[51] reported that FH_2-reductase and thymidine kinase activities were increased in vitamin B_{12}–deficient bone marrow cells and that these elevated activities fell to normal after treatment with vitamin B_{12}. The thymidine kinase activity decreased because of the normalization of *de novo* synthesis of thymine methyl groups that normally inhibit the enzyme activity. The decrease in thymidine kinase activity after the administration of vitamin B_{12} was believed to constitute further evidence of the inadequate synthesis of thymidine monophosphate from deoxyuridine monophosphate in pernicious anemia since the thymidine monophosphate formed in this pathway normally inhibits thymidine kinase. Bock et al.'s results are also consistent with the methyltetrahydrofolate trap hypothesis. Silber et al.[372] investigated ribonucleotide reductase activity in pernicious anemia, as did Metz et al.,[292] and concluded that the impaired DNA synthesis found in pernicious anemia or folate deficiency was not the result of decreased enzymatic activity of ribonucleotide reductase.

Recent studies of bone marrow cells from patients with coexisting iron deficiency and pernicious anemia have further elucidated the role of deoxyuridine in the biosynthesis of DNA in pernicious anemia and have suggested possible reasons why typical megaloblastic changes in erythroid precursors are masked when these two conditions coexist. Pedersen et al.[322] were the first to report that in patients with pernicious anemia who also had coexisting iron deficiency typical overt megaloblastic changes were not observed in the erythroid precursors. These changes became evident once the iron deficiency was treated. Van der Weyden et al.[408] subsequently utilized Killmann's observation[253] that preincubation of megaloblastic marrow with deoxyuridine failed to produce the normal suppression of tritiated thymidine uptake into DNA. However, after the addition of the iron chelating agent desferrioxamine to the cultures, both in pernicious anemia and folate deficiency, a partial correction of the impairment of the deoxyuridine suppression of tritiated thymidine uptake was noted.[408] The authors concluded that iron had a role in normal DNA synthesis.

Recently, Wickramasinghe and Longland[435] studied marrow erythroid cells from patients who were deficient in both vitamin B_{12} and iron. They found that these patients showed a normal incorporation of tritiated thymidine into DNA but that after iron therapy the mean rate of incorporation was depressed by 50%. These patients also showed a subnormal suppression of tritiated thymidine incorporation after incubation with deoxyuridine. After therapy with iron, this abnormality worsened. The authors postulated that the disturbance in DNA synthesis that occurred in vitamin B_{12} deficiency was ameliorated by the coexistence of iron deficiency.

Although the exact mechanisms for the masking effect of iron deficiency upon megaloblastic changes in pernicious anemia are unclear, several explanations for this phenomenon have been proposed.[408,435] In iron deficiency there may be increased amounts of deoxyuridine produced owing to decreased activity of the iron-dependent ribonucleoside diphosphate reductase, an enzyme responsible for the conversion of ribonucleotides to deoxyribonucleotides.[408] The increased amounts of deoxyuridine monophosphate thus produced might be converted to thymine DNA by nonenzymatic routes, thereby masking the typical megaloblastic changes in a patient who also had vitamin B_{12} deficiency. In these ways, it has been suggested that iron may play a role in DNA synthesis.

HISTONE ABNORMALITIES IN PERNICIOUS ANEMIA

Histones, basic nucleoproteins that bind DNA strands into compact masses of chromatin and are believed responsible for genetic replication and cellular differentiation, have been found to be abnormal in pernicious anemia. The suggestion that abnormalities in histones might be found in pernicious anemia was made in 1968 in a study that described a "clockface" chromatin pattern in pernicious anemia and folate-deficient megaloblasts,[238] as reproduced in Figure 96. Subsequent cytochemical studies[239] demonstrated that the nuclei

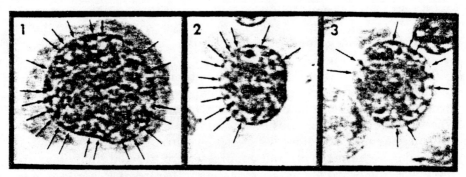

Figure 96. Clockface chromatin pattern (arrows) in fully developed megaloblasts (1) and in megaloblasts from minimally anemic patients (2 and 3). (From Blood 32:711, 1968. Reproduced with permission of Grune and Stratton, New York.)

of untreated pernicious anemia megaloblasts contained abundant lysine-rich histone and scant amounts of arginine-rich histone.

A recent study[240] investigated the biosynthesis of arginine-rich histones in pernicious anemia megaloblasts before and after treatment with vitamin B_{12} *in vivo* and *in vitro*. Using autoradiographic techniques, after exposure of these cells to vitamin B_{12}, a marked increase was seen in the concentration of tritium-labeled arginine in the nuclei of untreated pernicious anemia megaloblasts. Marked incorporation of both tritium-labeled lysine and especially tritium-labeled arginine into arginine-rich histone fractions was observed after exposure of the megaloblasts to vitamin B_{12}.

Coincident with the uptake of arginine that was interpreted as indicative of vitamin B_{12}–induced histone biosynthesis, there were differences observed in the electrophoretic patterns of both lysine- and arginine-rich histones obtained from megaloblasts before vitamin B_{12} treatment and from macronormoblasts after vitamin B_{12} treatment. Amino acid analyses of the histone fractions showed that the ratio of lysine to arginine was markedly decreased in the arginine-rich fractions after treatment with vitamin B_{12}, suggesting a substantial increase in the biosynthesis of arginine-rich histones.

In a subsequent study of histone abnormalities in pernicious anemia,[242] acetylation and methylation of histones were defective in untreated pernicious anemia megaloblasts. Acetylation and methylation were both markedly increased after exposure of the megaloblasts to vitamin B_{12} *in vivo* and *in vitro*. It was observed that the acetate moiety was incorporated directly into the histone molecule as a result of exposure of the histones to vitamin B_{12}. Moreover, it was found that the amino acid lysine, in particular, underwent methylation after exposure of histones to vitamin B_{12}.

GASTROINTESTINAL TRACT PATHOLOGY IN PERNICIOUS ANEMIA

Since the effects of vitamin B_{12} deficiency are widespread, it is not surprising that in pernicious anemia the cells of the gastrointestinal tract may demonstrate histological abnormalities. In some instances, these abnormalities are expressed as functional disturbances in the absorption of vitamin B_{12} (Chapter 6).

Farrant et al.[142] observed nuclear changes in the oral epithelium of patients with pernicious anemia. They studied 39 cases of pernicious anemia and noted that in the buccal mucosal cells there was a marked increase of the shorter axis of the nuclei. The nuclei appeared abnormally large in this axis, especially in untreated cases of pernicious anemia, and reverted to normal after therapy.

Graham et al.[174] found that there were characteristic cellular changes in gastric epithelial cells in pernicious anemia. They noted that squamous and columnar epithelial cells in untreated pernicious anemia were increased in size and that multinucleation was often seen. Rubin and Massey[356] reported that in patients with untreated pernicious anemia there were unique-appearing "PA" cells in the gastric mucosa. These were large gastric columnar cells with creased and folded nuclear membranes, vacuolated cytoplasm, and perinuclear haloes. The changes in these gastric cells were believed to be irreversible.

Sauli et al.[361] studied the histopathology of the small intestinal mucosa obtained by Crosby biopsy capsule in pernicious anemia before and after treatment with vitamin B_{12}. Before treatment some of the villi appeared normal, but others showed dendritic areas, fusion processes forming pseudocysts, and rare atrophy and diffuse round cell infiltration on the lamina propria. After treatment with vitamin B_{12}, these changes reverted to normal. Foroozan and Trier[151] also studied the histology of the small intestine in pernicious anemia. Before treatment with vitamin B_{12}, the villi appeared shortened with increased cells in the lamina propria. The cells were widened with large nuclei, and the intestinal cells contained Feulgen-positive bodies in their cytoplasm. Decreased mitoses were seen in intestinal crypts. These abnormalities disappeared after treatment with vitamin B_{12}.

CHAPTER 6

VITAMIN B$_{12}$

As a result of the pioneering studies of Rickes et al.,[345] Smith,[375,376,377] and Hodgkin et al.,[210-212] it is now known that vitamin B$_{12}$ is a cobalt-containing substance with molecular weight of 1355 and a formula of $C_{63}H_{88}O_{14}N_{14}PCo$. Diagrams of the formula of the vitamin B$_{12}$ molecule and its atomic configuration[52,206,332,373,442] are reproduced in Figure 97. In the cyanocobalamin molecule there are two portions. One is a nucleotide that lies almost perpendicular to a planar group. The second is the planar group that in some respects resembles the macro-ring of porphyrin. In the porphyrin portion of the cyanocobalamin molecule there are four reduced pyrrole rings that are linked to a central cobalt atom. A cyano group and a 5, 6-dimethylbenzimidazolyl group below the planar bridges occupy the two remaining positions.

Barker et al.[27] in 1958 discovered the biologically active form of vitamin B$_{12}$, designated as 5'-deoxyadenosylcobalamin or coenzyme B$_{12}$. This is presumed to be the form in which vitamin B$_{12}$ is hematopoietically active.[140,204] The formula and atomic configuration of coenzyme B$_{12}$ are shown in Figure 98. The deoxyadenosyl moiety of the coenzyme B$_{12}$ molecule is believed to be transferred directly to the vitamin from ATP by the action of a "coenzyme synthetase."[36]

Deoxyadenosylcobalamin aand methylcobalamin are the two currently known naturally occurring coenzymes of vitamin B$_{12}$. After exposure to light, both are oxidized to hydroxycobalamin.[206] Hydroxycobalamin is converted to the more stable compound cyanocobalamin in the presence of cyanide. Cyanocobalamin is the most commonly used pharmacological preparation of vitamin B$_{12}$ because of its stability. However, cyanocobalamin is metabolically inert and is probably converted by means as yet unknown to deoxyadenosylcobalamin within cells.[206] It has been proposed that this conversion takes place by means of a coenzyme synthetase system[36] in which ATP is the biological alkylating agent. The deoxyadenosyl moiety of the

149

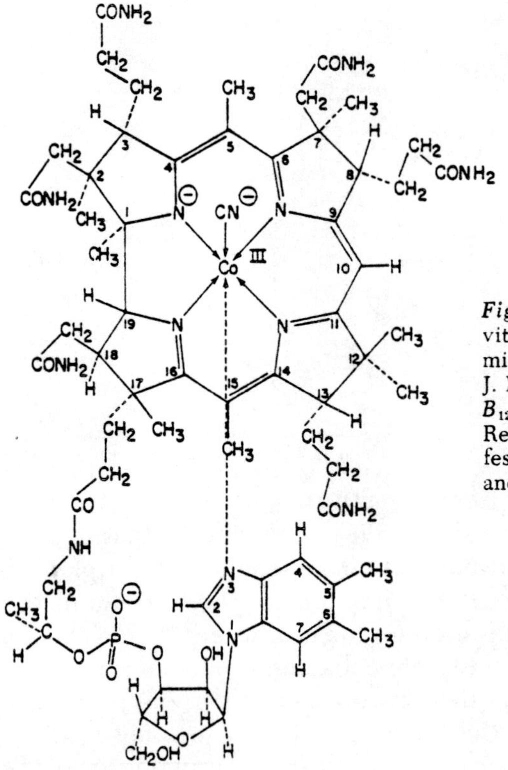

Figure 97. **A.** Structural formula of vitamin B$_{12}$. **B.** Spatial model of vitamin B$_{12}$ molecule. (*A* and *B* from Pratt, J. M. *Inorganic Chemistry of Vitamin B$_{12}$.* Academic Press, New York, 1972. Reproduced with permission of Professor J. M. Pratt, Johannesburg, S.A., and Academic Press, New York.)

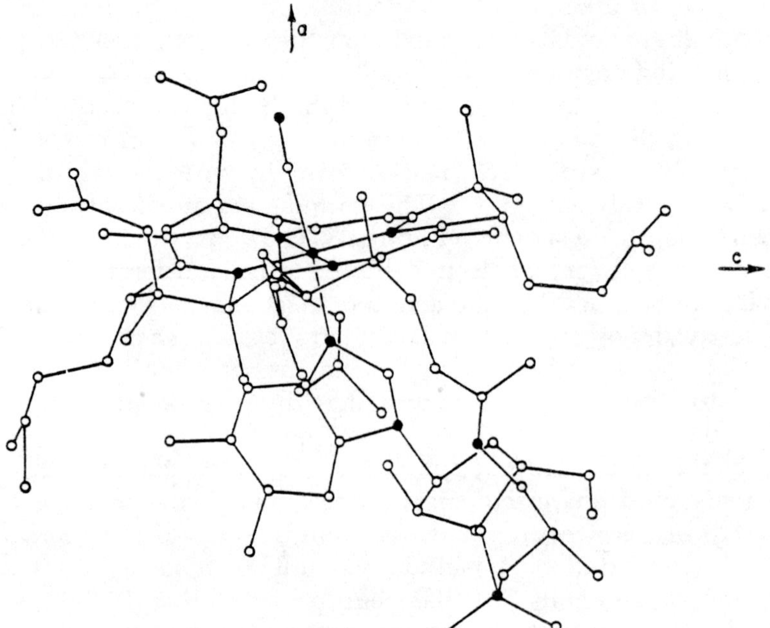

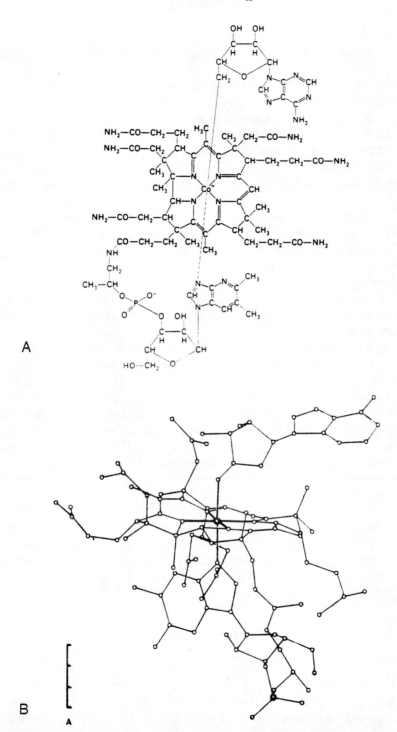

Figure 98. A. Structural formula of coenzyme B$_{12}$. (From *Biochemistry* by Stryer, L., W. H. Freeman and Company, San Francisco. Copyright © 1975.) *B.* Spatial model of coenzyme B$_{12}$ molecule. (From Fed. Proc. 23:594, 1964. Reproduced with permission of Professor Dorothy C. Hodgkin, Oxford, England, and Federation Proceedings.)

ATP molecule is transferred intact to the vitamin to form the coenzyme. The reaction also requires a reduced flavin or reduced ferredoxin, and a thiol or diol.

Most of the vitamin B$_{12}$ in plasma exists in the form of methylcobalamin, and coenzyme B$_{12}$ may be present in small amounts.[206] The normal body stores of vitamin B$_{12}$ have been estimated at between 3000 and 5000 micrograms, the majority of which is stored within the liver[88,403] in the form of coenzyme B$_{12}$. The kidneys are also believed to contain abundant amounts of coenzyme B$_{12}$.[36] Small amounts of methylcobalamin and hydroxycobalamin may also be stored in the liver.[206]

Vitamin B$_{12}$ is not synthesized within the gastrointestinal tract of humans nor is it available from green vegetables as is folate.[88] Vitamin B$_{12}$ is normally incorporated into the diet as a result of ingesting the flesh of ruminants such as cows or sheep. In contrast to man, these animals are capable of synthesizing vitamin B$_{12}$ within their gut as a result of bacterial action.[88,332] The cobalt contained in the vitamin B$_{12}$ molecule is present as a trace element in the pastures on which these ruminant animals graze.[283]

In most Western countries, the average diet contains 5-30 micrograms of vitamin B$_{12}$ daily, and approximately 1-5 micrograms/day are absorbed. Although the minimal effective daily dose requirement of vitamin B$_{12}$ has been estimated at 0.1 microgram/day,[388] the official United States Government recommended nutritional allowance is 5 micrograms per day.* Of an oral dose of 0.15-2.0 micrograms of vitamin B$_{12}$, approximately 60% to 80% is absorbed. However, the percent absorption of the vitamin actually decreases as the dose of oral vitamin B$_{12}$ increases, and at a dose of 5 micrograms, only 30% or less is absorbed. The amount of vitamin B$_{12}$ remaining after parenteral administration is governed by the availability of binding sites on the vitamin B$_{12}$ binding proteins, particularly transcobalamin I. In actual practice, if single parenteral doses of greater than 100 micrograms are given there may be insufficient binding sites for the vitamin on the carrier protein, and consequently the unbound vitamin B$_{12}$ may be lost through rapid renal excretion.

ABSORPTION OF VITAMIN B$_{12}$

Following entry into the gastrointestinal tract, vitamin B$_{12}$ is released from foodstuffs by the action of gastric proteolytic enzymes. Most of the vitamin then attaches to the glycoprotein intrinsic factor as a prerequisite to its absorption into the blood (Chapter 8). When the vitamin B$_{12}$–intrinsic factor complex reaches the sites of vitamin B$_{12}$

*Food and Nutrition Board, National Research Council: *Recommended Dietary Allowances*, 7th ed. No. 1964, National Academy of Sciences, Washington, D.C., 1968.

absorption on the brush borders of the epithelial cells of the terminal ileum,[54] a process of detachment of the vitamin from intrinsic factor occurs, and the vitamin is absorbed alone.[84-86,100,103,200,202,416] Intrinsic factor itself is not absorbed.[13,209,326] The intrinsic factor mechanism accounts for the majority of the vitamin B$_{12}$ absorbed. A much smaller amount, approximately 1% of free vitamin B$_{12}$, is passively absorbed throughout the small intestine, probably by diffusion.[203] The diffusion mechanism is believed to assume importance only in instances where vitamin B$_{12}$, designated as 5'-deoxyadenosylcobalamin or coenzyme normal diet.[103]

Laboratory Studies of Vitamin B$_{12}$ Absorption

Various authors have studied the mechanisms of vitamin B$_{12}$ absorption in the small intestine using *in vitro* systems. Strauss and Wilson[383] used sacs of everted small intestine incubated in a bicarbonate-saline mixture containing labeled vitamin B$_{12}$ with or without a source of intrinsic factor. They found that in both hamster and guinea pig the lowest part of the ileum was most active in vitamin B$_{12}$ uptake in the presence of intrinsic factor, and the upper jejunum showed little or no uptake. In their studies intrinsic factor did not bind to the intestine in the absence of vitamin B$_{12}$ even if calcium ions were present. They concluded that intrinsic factor and vitamin B$_{12}$ both had to be present to effect intestinal uptake of vitamin B$_{12}$.

Carmel et al.[77] studied vitamin B$_{12}$ uptake by human small bowel homogenates and its enhancement by intrinsic factor. They found that mucosal homogenates of human ileum showed enhanced vitamin B$_{12}$ uptake in the presence of normal human gastric juice or hog intrinsic factor concentrate. The uptake process required calcium and had a pH optimum at 6.6 and above. In contrast to the findings of others,[77,100,103,200,202,203,383,416] Highley and Ellenbogen[207] found that binding of intrinsic factor to vitamin B$_{12}$ was unnecessary for proper absorption of the vitamin and that vitamin B$_{12}$ did not preferentially bind to intrinsic factor.

Cooper and Castle[98] studied the sequential mechanisms by which intrinsic factor enhanced the absorption of vitamin B$_{12}$. They distinguished three phases of absorption. The first was a nonspecies related competitive binding of dietary vitamin B$_{12}$ by intrinsic factor. The second was a non-energy–requiring absorption of intrinsic factor–bound vitamin B$_{12}$ by intestinal mucosa involving bivalent cations, and the third was a species-related conversion of the calcium ion-dependent bond and release of free vitamin B$_{12}$ at the surface on or within the intestinal wall, possibly as a result of intestinal enzymatic action.

Autoradiographic studies using radioactive vitamin B$_{12}$ have provided further information regarding the sites of attachment of the vitamin to the intestinal epithelial cell and the mechanism of cellular transport during the process of absorption. Weisberg et al.[420] determined that ^{57}Co-B$_{12}$ two hours after administration was found in surface mucus contained in crypts and attached to villi and to mucin granules of goblet cells in both crypts and villi of dog intestinal cells. They concluded that the mucus of the goblet cell contained binders for vitamin B$_{12}$ that might facilitate the absorption of the vitamin.

Similar conclusions were reached by Donaldson et al.[119] who reported that hamster intrinsic factor markedly enhanced the uptake of ^{57}Co-cyanocobalamin by brush borders and microvillous membranes isolated from the distal intestinal villous epithelial cells of hamsters. Intrinsic factor–mediated attachment of ^{57}Co-B$_{12}$ to brush borders occurred rapidly, was not increased by removal of glucose or oxygen from the incubation medium, and was not decreased when the incubation temperature decreased from 37° to 7°C. A marked increase in uptake occurred in the absence of divalent cations. The authors suggested that there was a specific cellular receptor for the intrinsic factor–bound vitamin B$_{12}$.

The properties of this receptor for the vitamin B$_{12}$ –intrinsic factor complex in the ileal mucosa were studied by Rothenberg and Huhti.[354] They reported that immunologically intact intrinsic factor could be extracted from the ileum after *in vivo* incubation with a mixture of gastric juice and ^{57}Co-B$_{12}$ and that a macromolecular factor was present in the distal ileal mucosa that bound intrinsic factor *in vivo* and *in vitro*, changing its solubilities and electrophoretic properties. According to these authors, this ileal binding factor was the intestinal receptor for intrinsic factor. Using guinea pig ileal homogenates, Peters and Hoffbrand[326] reported that the vitamin B$_{12}$–intrinsic factor complex initially bound to a high molecular weight receptor (MW 100,000) on the brush border. After release of vitamin B$_{12}$ from intrinsic factor, the vitamin B$_{12}$ became attached to a lower molecular weight protein (MW 15,000-20,000) within the mucosa.

After binding to the intestinal receptors, the intrinsic factor–vitamin B$_{12}$ complex is then cleaved, perhaps in the ileal mucus on the brush border. The substance causing the release of vitamin B$_{12}$ from intrinsic factor in the ileum was studied by Highley et al.[208] These authors reported that the releasing substance was dialyzable and was localized in the proximal and mid-ileum of the rat small intestine. Non-radioactive vitamin B$_{12}$ was active in the release of bound radioactive vitamin B$_{12}$ and appeared to equilibrate with the bound form. The authors concluded that the releasing substance was actually endogenous vitamin B$_{12}$. Others[98] have suggested that the separation of vitamin B$_{12}$ from intrinsic factor may occur as the result of an enzymatic reaction.

Following disruption of the intrinsic factor–vitamin B$_{12}$ complex, vitamin B$_{12}$ alone enters the ileal epithelial cell. Cyanocobalamin, hydroxycobalamin, and coenzyme B$_{12}$ are all absorbed by the ileal cells, although coenzyme B$_{12}$ has been reported to be absorbed more slowly than cyanocobalamin,[204] suggesting that coenzyme B$_{12}$ must be converted to another form prior to absorption. Autoradiographic studies have shown that one hour following attachment of vitamin B$_{12}$ to the ileal mucus the vitamin appears in the underlying lamina propria, microvilli, terminal web, rough endoplasmic reticulum, Golgi complex, intercellular spaces, and capillaries of the lamina propria.[420]

Additional recent investigations of isolated subcellular components have shown that within the intestinal cell, vitamin B$_{12}$ is preferentially concentrated within the inner membranes of mitochondria. It has been suggested that the mitochondrion may be the major storage organelle for the vitamin in hepatic and ileal cells. The role of the mitochondrion in vitamin B$_{12}$ metabolism is unclear at present, but it has been hypothesized that the mitochondrion may carry vitamin B$_{12}$ through the cytoplasm of the ileal epithelial cell.[420]

Clinical Studies of Vitamin B$_{12}$ Absorption

Clinical studies of vitamin B$_{12}$ absorption have complemented developments in the understanding of the cellular mechanisms for absorption of this vitamin. Heinle et al.[198] were among the first to use radioisotopes in the evaluation of vitamin B$_{12}$ absorption in patients with pernicious anemia. Using ^{60}Co-B$_{12}$ they determined the degree of absorption of the labeled vitamin in patients with pernicious anemia by measuring with a scintillation counter the amount of radioactivity eliminated in the feces following the oral administration of small quantities (0.5 microgram) of the vitamin. They postulated that their method could be used to determine the potency of intrinsic factor preparations.

Booth and Mollin[53] found that when ^{56}Co-B$_{12}$ was given to normal persons, and to patients with untreated pernicious anemia, radioactivity was found in the plasma of pernicious anemia patients only if vitamin B$_{12}$ was given with intrinsic factor. The radioactivity appeared 3 to 6 hours after administration of the radioactive vitamin. The peak of the radioactivity occurred 8 to 12 hours after the dose. The amount of radioactive vitamin B$_{12}$ in the urine was greater in normals than in patients with pernicious anemia. Hepatic radioactivity rose slowly and peaked at two to six days. Glass[163] also studied the hepatic localization of vitamin B$_{12}$ and reported that radioactive B$_{12}$ concentrated in the liver and was stored there longer than in other organs. Approximately 95% of radioactive vitamin B$_{12}$ administered intramuscularly disappeared from the injection site within 2 hours and reached a peak in the liver in four to six days.

Another important study of vitamin B$_{12}$ absorption utilizing radioactive vitamin B$_{12}$ was reported by Schilling.[364] He found that when normal human gastric juice was given with radioactive vitamin B$_{12}$ to a patient with pernicious anemia there was increased excretion of radioactivity in the urine only if a "flushing" dose of nonradioactive vitamin B$_{12}$ was given. The flushing dose was 1000 micrograms of nonradioactive vitamin B$_{12}$ given intramuscularly. Schilling observed that there was no detectable radioactivity in the urine of pernicious anemia patients given ^{60}Co-B$_{12}$ alone, but radioactivity appeared if normal gastric juice was given. He postulated that when the non-radioactive vitamin B$_{12}$ was given intramuscularly (flushing dose), it saturated the plasma protein binding sites for vitamin B$_{12}$. Therefore, radioactive vitamin B$_{12}$ was not bound to protein, was cleared by the glomeruli, and appeared in the urine.

At the Simpson Memorial Institute, the University of Michigan Medical Center, and elsewhere, Schilling's observations have subsequently been utilized in the form of a test for the malabsorption of vitamin B$_{12}$. The Schilling test is performed in the following manner:

The patient must be fasting overnight and should not have received recent radioactivity. All parenteral vitamin preparations containing vitamin B$_{12}$ should be withheld for three days prior to the test, and on the day of the test, all oral vitamin preparations should be withheld. The collection of urine must be complete, since incomplete collections may lead to false positive results.

1. The patient is given a capsule containing 0.5 microcuries of ^{57}Co-B$_{12}$ by mouth. Two hours later, the patient is instructed to void. This sample of urine is discarded, and 1000 micrograms of nonradioactive cyanocobalamin are given intramuscularly. For the next 24 hours, all urine is saved and radioactivity measured.

2. If the results of the first part of the test are abnormal, a second test is performed that is identical to the first, except that 1 NF oral unit of intrinsic factor is given with the capsule of radioactive vitamin B$_{12}$.

Since the tests are predicated upon normal renal function, impaired renal function may alter the results. Particularly in the case of renal insufficiency, the urine collection may be extended to 72 hours and a flushing dose of 1000 micrograms of nonradioactive vitamin B$_{12}$ administered intramuscularly each day.

In typical pernicious anemia, less than 5% of administered radioactivity is recovered in the urine. Often it may be as small as 1% or less. After administration of intrinsic factor with the oral and flushing doses of vitamin B$_{12}$, the test usually normalizes, and greater than 5% of the radioactivity is detected. In some instances, ambiguous results are obtained in this second stage of the Schilling test, since patients with vitamin B$_{12}$ or folate deficiency may develop a secondary malabsorption syndrome. By treating the patient with vitamin B$_{12}$ and then repeating the study, the misleading results may then become clarified. Of course, if the amount of radioactivity recovered after the administration of intrinsic factor does not exceed 5%, it is also possible that an intestinal malabsorptive disorder unrelated to pernicious anemia or folate deficiency may be present. Thus, in cases of vitamin B$_{12}$ deficiency the use of the Schilling test first without and then with intrinsic factor may help to differentiate pernicious anemia from small intestinal disorders such as sprue, that may also cause malabsorption of vitamin B$_{12}$.

Clinical studies of vitamin B$_{12}$ absorption in disorders of the small intestine and in other conditions have also contributed to the knowledge concerning the site and mechanisms of vitamin B$_{12}$ absorption. Booth and Mollin[54] were the first to report that in patients whose ileum was resected, vitamin B$_{12}$ deficiency was often found, and therefore they implicated the ileum as the site of vitamin B$_{12}$ absorption. Cooper[101] extended Booth and Mollin's observations by reporting that most of the ^{60}Co-B$_{12}$ associated with the ileum during vitamin B$_{12}$ absorption in man was bound to material that had the properties of intrinsic factor. His findings helped to establish the intimate relationship between intrinsic factor and vitamin B$_{12}$ at the site of absorption. Doscherholmen and Hagen[121] found that five patients with portacaval shunts had delays in the peak of radioactivity consistent with slow absorption of vitamin B$_{12}$ from the intestine. They concluded that cyanocobalamin was temporarily stored in the intestinal wall.

Improvements in the intestinal malabsorptive defect of vitamin B$_{12}$ deficiency following the administration of vitamin B$_{12}$ have been noted by various authors. Schloesser and Schilling[366] studied an Asiatic Indian vegetarian who had defective absorption of vitamin B$_{12}$. Intrinsic factor was present in normal amounts in the patient's gastric juice. After treatment, the vitamin B$_{12}$ absorptive defect disappeared. Haurani et al.[192] also observed that in two patients with pernicious anemia there was malabsorption of the vitamin B$_{12}$–intrinsic factor complex that was corrected after administration of vitamin B$_{12}$.

Brody et al.[59] studied coexistent pernicious anemia and malabsorption in four patients. In nine consecutive patients with megaloblastic anemia and malabsorption including malabsorption for vitamin B$_{12}$, four had pernicious anemia with no demonstrable intrinsic factor. In these four patients, a generalized gastrointestinal malabsorptive defect was seen. The authors postulated that generalized malabsorption could occur coincident with small bowel lesions and be unrelated to the pernicious anemia. Carmel and Herbert[74] found that ten patients with pernicious anemia and no evidence of coincidental intestinal disease had intestinal malabsorption of vitamin B$_{12}$. This malabsorption was presumably related to abnormalities in the intestinal epithelial cells as a result of the vitamin B$_{12}$ deficiency.

In addition to the known associations between atrophic gastritis and pernicious anemia, abnormalities of vitamin B$_{12}$ absorption have also been reported following complete or partial surgical removal of the stomach and/or injury to the stomach.[10,115,186,278,281] Alsted[10] found that pernicious anemia developed in a 43-year-old woman 14 years after the ingestion of nitric acid. The corrosive action of the acid on the mucosa of the stomach was postulated as the pathogenetic factor in the development of pernicious anemia. MacDonald et al.[281] studied the late effects of total gastrectomy in man. Two of three patients developed macrocytic hyperchromic anemia 2 and 5 years respectively after gastrectomy. The other patient had received prophylactic injections of liver extract.

Lous and Schwartz[279] studied the absorption of vitamin B$_{12}$ following partial gastrectomy. They performed Schilling tests in 119 patients with partial gastrectomies performed six years prior to the study. Of 51 patients who had surgery for duodenal ulcers, 7 had abnormalities of vitamin B$_{12}$ absorption. Of 45 patients who had surgery for gastric ulcer, 5 had decreased vitamin B$_{12}$ absorption. In 17 patients who had surgery for carcinoma of the stomach, 13 had decreased absorption of vitamin B$_{12}$. The authors concluded that the risk of developing malabsorption of vitamin B$_{12}$ was greatest in patients who had surgery for carcinoma of the stomach.

Deller and Witts[115] also studied changes in serum vitamin B$_{12}$ levels following partial gastrectomy. In 265 patients 1 to 12 years after partial gastrectomy, vitamin B$_{12}$ deficiency was not rare. In 38 patients (14%) the serum vitamin B$_{12}$ level was below normal. Subnormal B$_{12}$ levels were seen after surgery when gastric ulcer was present, after the Polya type of operation, and if chronic gastritis was found in the resected stomach. Anemia was found in 54 patients (20.4%), and the serum iron was low in 34% of the patients.

TRANSPORT OF VITAMIN B$_{12}$

Following its passage through the intestinal epithelial cell, perhaps via the mitochondrion, vitamin B$_{12}$, primarily in the form of methylcobalamin, becomes bound to globulins in the blood. These proteins transport the vitamin to cells throughout the body.

Studies leading to the elucidation of the plasma transport mechanisms of vitamin B$_{12}$ had their beginnings in microbiological studies designed to measure the concentration of vitamin B$_{12}$ in the serum. In 1949, Hutner et al.[222] developed an assay of the "antipernicious anemia factor" using *Euglena gracilis*, a protozoan that has an absolute growth requirement for vitamin B$_{12}$. Ross also described an assay for vitamin B$_{12}$ in body fluids, using *E. gracilis*.[352,353] Lear et al.[266] found that in 33 patients with pernicious anemia using the *E. gracilis* method, the vitamin B$_{12}$ level was 39 picograms/milliliter or less, and no free vitamin B$_{12}$ was detected. *Lactobacillus leichmannii* is also used for the microbiological determination of vitamin B$_{12}$ and is thought to be more rapid than the *E. gracilis* technique.[36] Although accurate radioimmunoassays for vitamin B$_{12}$ using coated charcoal have been developed,[251] at present the microbiological methods are used most frequently.

Evidence of vitamin B$_{12}$ binding proteins initially appeared in the studies of Pitney et al., [328] who were the first to report that vitamin B$_{12}$ existed in serum largely in a bound form. They found that alpha-globulins in particular were the specific serum protein fractions in which most of the vitamin B$_{12}$ was located. Beard et al.[29] observed that the vitamin B$_{12}$ level in chronic granulocytic leukemia was fifteen times normal and was normal in chronic lymphocytic leukemia. They explained this striking increase in chronic granulocytic leukemia by noting that the vitamin B$_{12}$ in this disorder was bound to increased amounts of vitamin B$_{12}$–binding proteins. Miller and Sullivan[293] found that both the α_1-globulin and β-globulin were capable of binding vitamin B$_{12}$, and that the vitamin B$_{12}$ binding capacity was markedly elevated in chronic granulocytic leukemia, explaining the marked elevation of serum vitamin B$_{12}$ in this disorder.

Mendelsohn et al.[289] found that vitamin B$_{12}$ was bound primarily to an α_1-globulin in both normal persons and in patients with chronic granulocytic leukemia. The B$_{12}$ binding protein they described is believed to carry the vitamin in the plasma for an extended period of time and was subsequently called transcobalamin I.[182,184] Miller and Sullivan[294] separated vitamin B$_{12}$ binding protein from other serum proteins by electrophoresis in starch gel at pH 4.5. They found that the vitamin B$_{12}$–binding protein was in the seromucoid fraction and was a protein with the mobility of the α_1-glycoproteins at pH 4.5. The protein was not precipitated with Cohen fraction VI. Weinstein et al.[419] also observed that ^{58}Co-B$_{12}$ localized in the seromucoid fraction of plasma and that the vitamin B$_{12}$ binding protein was a glycoprotein.

The initial observation that there may be more than one vitamin B$_{12}$–binding protein was made by Hall and Finkler.[180] They found that injected vitamin B$_{12}$ was bound to more than one plasma fraction. The disappearance of vitamin B$_{12}$ from each fraction took place at different rates. In vitamin B$_{12}$–deficient patients, most of the vitamin B$_{12}$ was localized in the fractions with the slower rate of vitamin B$_{12}$ loss. Shortly after the detection of these two fractions, Hall and Finkler[181] were able to characterize more fully a vitamin B$_{12}$–binding protein separate from the α_1-globulin identified earlier by Mendelsohn et al.[289] This newly identified protein was believed to "function at an earlier stage of distribution of vitamin B$_{12}$ than the α_1-globulin, and it may prove to be important in the movement of vitamin B$_{12}$ from the intestine to tissue." Hall and Finkler called this transport protein transcobalamin II[182] to distinguish it from the α_1-globulin vitamin

B$_{12}$–binding protein identified earlier,[289] which they called trans-cobalamin I.

Transcobalamin II was found to function in the transport of vitamin B$_{12}$ shortly after intake into the body, and vitamin B$_{12}$ bound to transcobalamin II was found to disappear rapidly from plasma.[181,183,184] Transcobalamin II was found to be a β-globulin and appeared to have "some intrinsic factor activity" although there was no evidence to suggest that it was circulating intrinsic factor. Transcobalamin II was also found to be the dominant binder of recently ingested and absorbed vitamin B$_{12}$ and had a molecular weight of less than 40,000. The unsaturated binding capacity of transcobalamin II in normal plasma ranges from 600 to 1500 picograms/milliliter.

Transcobalamin I, on the other hand, identified earlier by Mendelsohn[289] as an α_1-globulin, was believed to function in the transport of endogenous vitamin B$_{12}$ and apparently to be the major B$_{12}$-binding protein in plasma. Normally, more than half of the binding capacity of transcobalamin I is saturated with vitamin B$_{12}$. In pernicious anemia, the binding capacity of transcobalamin I is undersaturated. Recent studies[103] have suggested that transcobalamin I may be derived in part from granulocytes. Vitamin B$_{12}$ bound to transcobalamin I in both normal persons and patients with chronic granulocytic leukemia disappeared from plasma at a much slower rate than vitamin B$_{12}$ bound to transcobalamin II.[182,184]

ENTRY OF VITAMIN B$_{12}$ INTO CELLS

After vitamin B$_{12}$ reaches the cells by way of the plasma transport globulins, it attaches to and then enters these cells. Various studies have examined the mechanisms by which this attachment and entry occur. Cooper and Paranchych[99] found that mouse ascitic fluid and human serum caused a 20-fold increase in the uptake of vitamin B$_{12}$ by mouse ascitic cells and HeLa cells, indicating that there was a selective uptake of specifically bound cobalt-labeled vitamin B$_{12}$ by human and mouse tumor cells. Paranchych and Cooper[319] reported that the uptake of cyanocobalamin by Ehrlich ascitic carcinoma cells was biphasic. There was a primary rapid phase and a secondary slower phase. The primary phase was the uptake part of the biphasic process. It was believed to represent a physiochemical reaction between extracellularly-bound cyanocobalamin and receptors on the cell membrane. The secondary uptake phase was believed to involve the transport of cyanocobalamin from the receptors to the cell. The primary phase was not affected by variations in temperature, pH, and cellular energy. The secondary phase, however, was optimal at pH 7.4 and was sensitive to variations in temperature and to various metabolic inhibitors. According to these authors, the primary uptake phase was the uptake-limiting step of the overall uptake process.

The uptake of vitamin B$_{12}$ into the erythrocyte was described by Retief et al.[344] They studied serum-mediated ^{57}Co-B$_{12}$ uptake by reticulocyte-rich erythrocyte suspensions and found that rapid adsorption of the radioactive vitamin B$_{12}$ to the erythrocyte surface occurred. Ionic calcium and magnesium were required, although strontium could partially replace these ions. The uptake increased during a rising reticulocyte count. Trypsin and papain decreased the uptake. EDTA (ethylenediamine tetraacetic acid) could elute all of the vitamin B$_{12}$ adsorbed to the surface of the erythrocyte. The authors postulated that there were two mechanisms for vitamin B$_{12}$ adsorption to the surface of the erythrocyte: (1) calcium or magnesium-dependent, carrier, glycoprotein mediated transfer to receptors on the cell surface, operative primarily in the presence of physiological amounts of vitamin B$_{12}$, and (2) simple diffusion independent of the receptor sites, primarily operative in the presence of excess unbound vitamin B$_{12}$.

Herbert and Sullivan[204] found that human reticulocytes showed a greater uptake of coenzyme B$_{12}$ than cyanocobalamin from plasma. They suggested that the reticulocytes possessed specific receptor sites for coenzyme B$_{12}$. It was also found that an *in vivo* bolus of coenzyme B$_{12}$ entered the interior of the cells at a slower rate than a comparable bolus of cyanocobalamin, perhaps indicating that coenzyme B$_{12}$ had to be converted to another form prior to passage through the cell membrane into the cell.

MECHANISM OF ACTION OF VITAMIN B$_{12}$ IN MAN

A number of studies have been performed to elucidate the mechanism of action of vitamin B$_{12}$, and particularly the relationships between vitamin B$_{12}$ and folate in pernicious anemia. Early experiments by Bennett et al.[39] helped to establish that vitamin B$_{12}$ was essential for normal growth. They found that crystalline vitamin B$_{12}$, vitamin B$_{12}$ contained in liver, or animal protein enabled rats to develop normally and to maintain normal livers on a labile-methyl-free homocysteine diet containing folic acid. Relationships between vitamin B$_{12}$ and folate were also explored initially by Bethell et al.[43] who reported that normal individuals could convert the conjugated form of folate to the free form, but patients with untreated pernicious anemia could not. In contrast to patients with untreated pernicious anemia, normal individuals excreted large amounts of pteroylglutamate.

These early observations indicating a close metabolic relationship between vitamin B$_{12}$ and folate were subsequently extended and clarified by Herbert and Zalusky.[201] They demonstrated that in pernicious anemia, pteroylglutamic acid was rapidly converted, probably to N-methyltetrahydrofolic acid. This substance then "accumulated" in the serum since vitamin B$_{12}$ was believed to be required for its normal utilization. Zalusky and Herbert[445] also found that a metabolic relationship existed between vitamin B$_{12}$ and folate in the case of formiminoglutamic acid. This metabolite was originally reported to be increased in the urine after a histidine load only in the case of folate deficiency.[390] Zalusky and Herbert,[445] however, found that for- miminoglutamicaciduria occurred in both vitamin B$_{12}$ and folate deficiency and was not specific for folate deficiency as originally thought.

These indications that there were closely related abnormalities of both folate and vitamin B$_{12}$ metabolism in pernicious anemia were studied at length by others.[161,283,311,422] On the basis of these and their own studies, Buchanan,[61,62] Noronha and Silverman[313] and Herbert and Zalusky[201] have advanced the *methyltetrahydrofolate trap* hypothesis to explain the interrelationships between vitamin B$_{12}$ and folate metabolism in pernicious anemia. This hypothesis, reviewed by Buchanan,[62] Johns and Bertino,[229] and others,[206,373] states that most of the metabolic effects of vitamin B$_{12}$ are mediated through folate.

According to the trap hypothesis, the methylcobalamin- dependent methyltransferase enzyme is required to convert methyl- tetrahydrofolate into other folate derivatives. In vitamin B$_{12}$ deficien- cy, the activity of this methyltransferase is significantly diminished. Because of this enzymatic abnormality, methyltetrahydrofolate ac- cumulates at the expense of other folates. As a consequence of the decrease in tetrahydrofolate, 5,10-methylenetetrahydrofolate, and formyltetrahydrofolate, the rates of reactions that are dependent upon these folate coenzymes are slowed. Ultimately DNA synthesis is re- tarded, resulting in megaloblastosis.

In support of the trap hypothesis, a direct role for vitamin B$_{12}$ in DNA synthesis has not as yet been demonstrated.[19,206,373] More direct evidence obtained by several authors also appears to have substan- tiated certain aspects of the trap hypothesis. Nixon and Bertino[312] found that in patients with untreated pernicious anemia, serum clear- ance rates of tracer doses of tritiated 5-methyltetrahydrofolate were markedly decreased. After treatment with vitamin B$_{12}$, the serum clearance rates of labeled 5-methyltetrahydrofolate became normal, indicating that proper utilization of this substance required a cobala- min. Additional evidence supporting the trap hypothesis was reported recently by Taylor et al.,[396] who demonstrated that a methyl- cobalamin-dependent methyltetrahydrofolate-homocysteine methyl- transferase could be detected in homogenates of normal bone mar- rows. In homogenates of marrow from a patient with untreated per- nicious anemia, methyltransferase activity as reflected by generation of radiolabeled methionine was very low, but increased markedly after the addition of methylcobalamin. Their report indicated that in untreated pernicious anemia marrow, the methyltransferase enzyme existed primarily in the apoenzyme form lacking the methylcobalamin prosthetic group. Objections to the methyltetrahydrofolate trap hypothesis have been discussed by Nixon and Bertino[311] and by Chanarin.[89] Metabolic consequences of abnormalities of the two vitamin B$_{12}$–dependent enzymes identified thus far in man are discussed in Chapters 7 and 10.

SUMMARY

Vitamin B$_{12}$ is a cobalt-containing substance with molecular weight of 1355 and a formula of C$_{63}$H$_{88}$O$_{14}$N$_{14}$PCo. It is synthesized by bacteria in the gut of ruminants. The normal body stores of vitamin B$_{12}$ range between 3000 and 5000 micrograms, and most of the vitamin is stored in the liver in the form of coenzyme B$_{12}$. The minimum effective daily adult dose requirement of vitamin B$_{12}$ is 0.1 microgram/day.[388] With this dose, a slight reticulocytosis accompanied by rise in hemoglobin and hematocrit is seen in untreated pernicious anemia patients. Despite this hematopoietic response, at the 0.1 microgram dose level the marrow remains megaloblastic, and elevations in serum B$_{12}$ levels and decreases in serum iron concentrations are not seen.[388] The official U.S. Government recommended nutritional allowance of vitamin B$_{12}$ is 5 micrograms per day.

The biologically active form of the vitamin is known as coenzyme B$_{12}$, or 5′-deoxyadenosylcobalamin. Hematopoietically at the 0.1 microgram/day dose level in untreated pernicious anemia, coenzyme B$_{12}$ is more active than cyanocobalamin.[388] In man coenzyme B$_{12}$ functions as a prosthetic group in the enzyme methylmalonyl-CoA mutase. This enzyme is responsible for the conversion of L-methylmalonyl-CoA to succinyl-CoA. The methylated form of vitamin B$_{12}$, or methyl-cobalamin, functions as a prosthetic group in the enzyme N^5-methyltetrahydrofolate-homocysteine methyltransferase. This enzyme is involved in the methylation of homocysteine to form methionine.

Upon entry into the gastrointestinal tract, vitamin B$_{12}$ is released from foodstuffs, and most of it becomes avidly bound to the glycoprotein, intrinsic factor. In the terminal ileum there are specific receptor sites for the vitamin B$_{12}$–intrinsic factor complex. Bivalent cations, particularly calcium, are involved in the adsorption of the intrinsic factor—B$_{12}$ complex to the surface mucous receptors. The absorptive are probably glycoproteins or mucopolysaccharides,[103] and are capable of binding the intrinsic factor-B$_{12}$ complex. The absorptive process is active and requires a pH optimum of 6.6 or above. The absorption is blocked by antibodies to intrinsic factor. Finally, in an as yet undefined manner and possibly as a result of an enzymatic reaction, free vitamin B$_{12}$ is released from intrinsic factor at the surface of or within the intestinal wall. It is believed by some that the releasing substance may be endogenous vitamin B$_{12}$. Intrinsic factor itself is not absorbed into the epithelial cell and does not enter the blood.[209] The vitamin B$_{12}$ subsequently enters the ileal mucosal cell where it is concentrated within mitochondria.

Most of the vitamin B$_{12}$ in the blood exists in the form of methyl-cobalamin, bound by two plasma proteins that transport it to the tissues. The α_1-globulin known as transcobalamin I is involved in the transport of endogenous vitamin B$_{12}$. The β-globulin, transcobalamin II, with molecular weight of less than 40,000, binds the newly absorbed vitamin B$_{12}$.

The uptake of vitamin B$_{12}$ by cells is believed to be a biphasic process. In the case of erythrocytes, rapid adsorption of the vitamin to the surface of the erythrocyte occurs. Presumably, hydroxycobalamin, methylcobalamin, and cyanocobalamin are converted to the biologically active form, coenzyme B$_{12}$, in a manner as yet unknown,[206] but perhaps as a result of a "coenzyme synthetase" reaction involving ATP.[36]

The pathophysiological basis for the biochemical abnormalities in vitamin B$_{12}$ deficiency is not fully understood. The abnormalities are believed by some to be mediated via folate and to be explainable on the basis of a methyltetrahydrofolate trap. According to this hypothesis, a decrease in the methylcobalamin-dependent methyltransferase enzyme leads to a deficit of folate metabolites that ultimately causes a decrease in the synthesis of thymine DNA, resulting in megaloblastosis.

CHAPTER 7

VITAMIN B$_{12}$–DEPENDENT ENZYMES IN MAN

Although a number of enzymes have been found to be vitamin B$_{12}$–dependent in bacteria and in lower animals,[332,373] to date there have been only two vitamin B$_{12}$–dependent enzymes isolated in man. These are the methylcobalamin-dependent enzyme N^5-methyltetrahydrofolate-homocysteine methyltransferase, and the 5'-deoxyadenosylcobalamin–dependent enzyme methylmalonyl-CoA mutase.[373] Because of their possible pathogenetic relationships to pernicious anemia, these two enzymes will be discussed in detail.

N^5-METHYLTETRAHYDROFOLATE-HOMOCYSTEINE METHYLTRANSFERASE

This enzyme that contains methylcobalamin as a prosthetic group catalyzes the formation of methionine from homocysteine and is believed to be important in the generation of methionine for other biosynthetic processes.[116,154,373] The activity of this enzyme is reduced in vitamin B$_{12}$–deficient animals.[116,256,373] Very recently, Taylor et al.[396] were the first to report that a methylcobalamin-dependent N^5-methyltetrahydrofolate-homocysteine methyltransferase could be detected in extracts of human bone marrows. In one case of severe untreated pernicious anemia, they found that the generation of radiolabeled methionine was markedly reduced compared to normal controls. After addition of methylcobalamin to the pernicious anemia marrow extract, methionine generation increased almost eightfold, demonstrating that in vitamin B$_{12}$–deficient bone marrow, methyltransferase exists predominantly in the form of an apoenzyme lacking the methylcobalamin prosthetic group. The reaction catalyzed by this

165

methylcobalamin-dependent methyltransferase enzyme is diagrammed as follows:

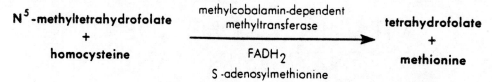

Early experiments on transmethylation by du Vigneaud et al.[124] in 1939 demonstrated that homocysteine could not replace methionine in the diet of the white rat supplemented with other B factors known or unrecognized at the time. Growth did occur when methionine was replaced by homocysteine *and* choline. Their work demonstrating that methionine could be formed by transfer of a methyl group of choline to homocysteine established the concept of biological transmethylation. Later, Moyer and du Vigneaud[302] studied the structural specificity of choline and betaine in the process of transmethylation. They found that in rats fed a diet containing homocysteine but lacking methionine, only choline, lecithin, phosphocholine, betaine, and dimethylethylhydroxyethylammonium chloride could act as methyl donors.

Subsequently, Davis and Mingioli[112] studied mutants of *Escherichia coli* that required methionine or vitamin B$_{12}$. They determined that these B$_{12}$-requiring mutants accumulated a precursor of methionine that was capable of sustaining the homocysteineless mutants. The mutants requiring vitamin B$_{12}$ or methionine did not respond to homocysteine, the immediate precursor of methionine. Also the mutants responding to homocysteine did not require vitamin B$_{12}$. The authors concluded that vitamin B$_{12}$ was concerned with the methylation of methionine.

Hatch et al.[191] then identified three essential enzymatic fractions involved in the biosynthesis of the methyl group of methionine in *E. coli*. One factor was a serine hydroxymethylase. A second factor was an enzyme that had a vitamin B$_{12}$ prosthetic group. A third fraction contained a third enzyme that was lacking in a methionine-requiring mutant strain of *E. coli*. A combination of these three enzyme fractions in the presence of required cofactors, substrates, and anaerobic conditions was capable of promoting methionine synthesis. There was also an absolute requirement for serine, homocysteine, pyridoxal phosphate, THFA, ATP, DPNH, FAD, or FMN. Subsequent studies by Larrabee et al.[262,263] and by Guest et al.[178,179] established that the methyl donor for methionine formation was methyltetrahydrofolate and that it was required in stoichiometric amounts.

Takeyama et al.[392] also found that there was an essential enzyme involved in the biosynthesis of the methyl group of methionine in Strain 113-3 of *E. coli*. This enzyme contained a derivative of vitamin

B$_{12}$ as a prosthetic group. The optimal formation of the vitamin B$_{12}$ enzyme from its apoenzyme and vitamin B$_{12}$ was obtained by incubation of tetrahydrofolate, FAD, ATP, and magnesium ions.

Guest et al.[178] studied a methyl analogue of cobamide coenzymes in relation to methionine synthesis by bacteria. They found that when homocysteine was incubated in a medium containing methylcobalamin there was a slow generation of methionine. The methyl group transferred to the homocysteine was the one limited to the cobalt and not one of those present as side groups on the corrin ring. They were able to make this assumption since hydroxycobalamin was inactive in the reaction. The authors believed that methylcobalamin might have been a transient compound in this reaction.

Foster et al.[153,154] found that the cobalamin of the vitamin B$_{12}$ enzyme had to be reduced by FADH$_2$ before the enzyme could catalyze the transfer of methyl groups from the N^5-methyltetrahydrofolic acid to homocysteine in the presence of S-adenosylmethionine. They postulated that S-adenosylmethionine acted as a catalyst. The isolated enzyme was reduced by FADH$_2$ and combined with S-adenosylmethionine. Methylcobalamin was then formed directly on the enzyme itself. The S-adenosyl-L-homocysteine thus produced on the enzyme was methylated by N^5-methyltetrahydrofolic acid so that when the methyl group of the cobalamin was transferred to homocysteine, S-adenosylmethionine was immediately available to remethylate the unstable vitamin B$_{12}$.

Loughlin et al.[278] were able to isolate a cobalamin-containing transmethylase (the N^5-methyltetrahydrofolate-homocysteine transmethylase) from mammalian liver. They found that magnesium ions were required as cofactors, as were FADH$_2$ and S-adenosylmethionine. 5-Methyltetrahydropteroyl monoglutamate was the substrate for the methyltransferase reaction in pig liver, and S-adenosylmethionine was the catalyst. The transmethylase enzyme contained a methylcobalamin prosthetic group.

Weissbach et al.[421] found that methyl-, ethyl-, and beta-propionate B$_{12}$ could transfer the methyl group from N^5-methyltetrahydrofolic acid to homocysteine. Taylor and Weissbach[394] reported that ^{14}C-methylmethionine was identified as the radioactive transmethylation produced from N^5[^{14}C]methyltetrahydrofolate when unlabeled methyl iodide was substituted for S-adenosylmethionine in the reduced flavin mononucleotide system. The authors concluded that S-adenosylmethionine activated the vitamin B$_{12}$ enzyme by methylation. A reactive methyl or ethyl group structure appeared to be the essential feature for S-adenosylmethionine cofactor activity.

Taylor and Weissbach[395] also studied the formation and photolability of a methylcobalamin-dependent methyltransferase isolated from *E. coli*. When they added reduced *E. coli* vitamin B$_{12}$ transmethylase to N^5[^{14}C]methyltetrahydrofolate, unlabeled S-adenosylmethionine, and S-adenosyl-L-[methyl-^{14}C]methionine alone or with methyl-^{14}C, methyl-^{14}C-cobalamin enzyme was formed. This enzyme was stable in the presence of light at 0° C unless the protein solution was acidified to pH 2.0.

Waxman et al.[416] determined that in bone marrow from vitamin B$_{12}$–deficient subjects DNA synthesis was abnormally reduced. They found that this inadequate DNA synthesis was due to a block in tetrahydrofolate regeneration from 5-methyltetrahydrofolate via homocysteine methylation. In their studies they measured the ability of deoxyuridine to suppress ^{3}H thymidine uptake in DNA. They observed that homocysteine facilitated and methionine reduced *de novo* DNA synthesis. The homocysteine effect in vitamin B$_{12}$–deficient marrow was believed to indicate that, in man, there was an additional vitamin B$_{12}$–dependent pathway for the regeneration of tetrahydrofolic acid. They explained the inhibitory effect of methionine by suggesting that there was an end-product inhibition of homocysteine transmethylase reaction, resulting in further accumulation of 5-methyltetrahydrofolic acid. Waxman et al. stated that homocysteine transmethylation might be critical in regulating the amount of available tetrahydrofolic acid and subsequent *de novo* synthesis of DNA.

METHYLMALONYL-CoA MUTASE

This enzyme, containing coenzyme vitamin B$_{12}$ (5'-deoxyadenosylcobalamin) as a prosthetic group, converts L-methylmalonyl-CoA to succinyl-CoA by a process of isomerization.[170,373] It is involved in the propionate metabolic pathway, and its position and mode of action are diagrammed opposite. Methylmalonyl-CoA mutase is believed to be localized almost exclusively in the inner membranes and matrices of mitochondria.*

Initially, Eggerer et al.[126,127] were the first to report that the isomerization of methylmalonyl-CoA to succinyl-CoA catalyzed by extracts of *Propionibacterium shermanii* was dependent on coenzyme B$_{12}$. In the course of the reaction, 2-^{14}C-methylmalonyl-CoA was converted to 3-^{14}C-succinyl-CoA. The isomerization was believed to occur by a shift of the thioester group. Isomerization occurred by a radical reaction mechanism involving an oxyreduction between substrate and enzyme. Lengyel et al.[269] later isolated methylmalonyl isomerase apoenzyme from sheep kidney cortex. The activity of the apoenzyme was restored by dimethylbenzimidazolyl and benzimidazolylcobalamide, both of which were the vitamin B$_{12}$ prosthetic groups of the enzyme.

Cox and White[107] made the first clinical observation of the role of methylmalonic acid in pernicious anemia by discovering that urinary

---

*Frenkel, E. P., Kitchens, R. L., Srere, P. A., and Orici, L. Mitochondrial alterations in vitamin B$_{12}$ deprivation in animals and man. Reported to the American Society of Hematology in Atlanta, Georgia, December, 1974.

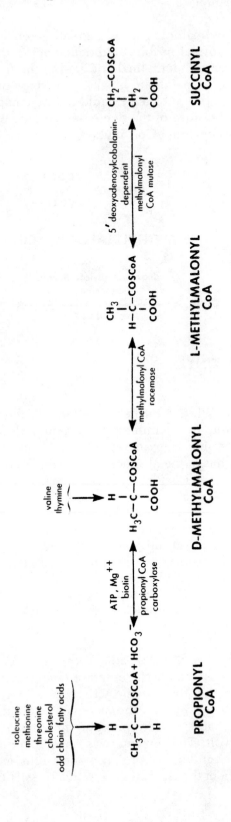

excretion of methylmalonic acid was greatly increased in pernicious anemia but was normal in folic acid deficiency and low in iron deficiency. The increased methylmalonic acid in the urine was believed to be the result of a metabolic block at the stage of methylmalonyl-CoA. Presumably, this substance could not be completely converted to succinyl-CoA because of the decreased activity of the vitamin B$_{12}$-dependent methylmalonyl-CoA mutase.

$$CH_3-CH \Big\langle {}^{COOH}_{COOH}$$

METHYLMALONIC ACID

$$H-\underset{\underset{COOH}{|}}{\overset{\overset{CH_3}{|}}{C}}-COSCoA \xleftrightarrow[\text{methylmalonyl CoA mutase}]{\substack{\text{deoxyadenosylcobalamin-}\\ \text{dependent}}} \underset{\underset{COOH}{|}}{\overset{\overset{CH_2-COSCoA}{|}}{CH_2}}$$

**L-METHYLMALONYL   SUCCINYL
CoA   CoA**

    Arnstein and White[19] further investigated abnormalities in the propionate pathway by examining the function of vitamin B$_{12}$ in the metabolism of propionate by the protozoan *Ochromonas malhamensis*. They found that in the absence of vitamin B$_{12}$ there was virtually a complete block in the oxidation of propionate that was corrected by the addition of cyanocobalamin.

    Wood et al.[441] reviewed the role of methylmalonyl-CoA and concluded that in the conversion of succinyl-CoA to methylmalonyl-CoA, the carbonyl thioester group was transferred and the free carbonyl group was not transferred. They believed that this was an intramolecular conversion. The transfer of hydrogen was not considered to involve a free proton. A proton was taken up in the conversion of the *a* isomer of methylmalonyl-CoA to succinyl-CoA, but this occurred during the racemization of methylmalonyl-CoA to the *b* isomer by a racemase enzyme.

    Kellermeyer et al.[250] were able to purify and characterize the properties of a methylmalonyl isomerase obtained from propionibacteria. They found that the specific activity was 14.4, the enzyme was colorless, the S20, w=7.0, and the molecular weight was 56,000. The purified enzyme had an electrophoretic mobility of 14.6×10^{-2} cm^2 per second per volt. The enzyme was not dependent on sulfhydryl groups for activity and did not require potassium or ammonium ions. EDTA did not affect the isomerase activity. The pH optimum was 7.4.

The Km for succinyl-CoA and methylmalonyl-CoA were 3.45 ×10^{-5} and 8 ×10^{-5} respectively.

Cannata et al.[71] also purified a methylmalonyl-CoA mutase from animal tissue. Using sheep liver as the source, they obtained the holoenzyme of methylmalonyl-CoA mutase approximately 7000-fold purified. The sedimentation coefficient was 7.75, the molecular weight was 165,000, and it had one mole of cobamide coenzyme per 75,000 grams, or roughly two moles per mole of enzyme. The K′ values (succinyl-CoA/L-methylmalonyl-CoA) was 18.6. D-methylmalonyl-CoA inhibited the isomerization of L-methylmalonyl-CoA. The apoenzyme was inactive, but full activity could be restored by adding the DBC enzyme. The holoenzyme was very stable, but the apoenzyme was unstable, especially in solutions of low ionic strength. The enzyme was stabilized in the presence of glutathione or cobamide coenzyme. The holoenzyme was resistant, and the apoenzyme was sensitive to sulfhydryl binding reagents.

Retey et al.[343] found that the methylmalonyl-CoA reaction involved an intermolecular transfer of hydrogen. They diagrammed the reaction as follows.

(in methylmalonyl CoA)   (in succinyl CoA)

Abeles and Zabalak[1] determined that the hydrogen that was removed from the C-1 of a particular diol during the conversion to the corresponding aldehyde was not necessarily the same hydrogen that replaced the hydroxyl group of the diol. They therefore concluded that the conversion of L-methylmalonyl-CoA to succinyl-CoA did not necessarily involve an intramolecular reaction. Cardinale and Abeles[73] found that in the reaction catalyzed by methylmalonyl-CoA mutase, the hydrogen was transferred from the C-5′ position of the coenzyme to the substrate as in the reaction catalyzed by dioldehydrase.

Frey et al.[156] reported that when [^{3}H]dl-1,2-propanediol was converted to propionaldehyde in the presence of dioldehydrase and cobamide coenzyme, the tritium label was transferred to the coenzyme. The coenzyme was tritiated solely in the C-5′ position of the adenosyl moiety. This represented an inter- and intramolecular transfer of the tritiated hydrogen. The hydrogen was abstracted from C-1 of dl-1,2-propanediol and transferred to the coenzyme where it became equivalent with at least one, but probably both, hydrogens of the C-5′

position. This led to the formation of a reduced fórm of the coenzyme and a molecule derived from the oxidation of the substrate. In a subsequent step, the hydrated form of propionaldehyde was formed by the transfer of hydrogen from reduced coenzyme to the intermediate derived from the substrate.

SUMMARY

Vitamin B$_{12}$ has been shown to participate in a number of biological reactions in bacteria and in lower animals. Thus far in man, only two enzymes have been found to be vitamin B$_{12}$–dependent. One of these is the methylcobalamin-dependent N^5-methyltetrahydrofolate-homocysteine methyltransferase. This enzyme catalyzes the methylation of homocysteine by the methyl group of methyltetrahydrofolate, to form methionine. Cofactors essential for this reaction include FADH$_2$ and S-adenosylmethionine. S-adenosylmethionine is believed to remethylate the unstable vitamin B$_{12}$ during the reaction. The *methyltetrahydrofolate trap* hypothesis is based upon the presumption that with a deficit in methyltransferase, methyltetrahydrofolate and other metabolites accumulate. This is believed to lead ultimately to a decrease in the synthesis of purines and pyrimidines dependent on various forms of folate and a net decrease in the synthesis of thymine DNA resulting in megaloblastosis.

The second vitamin B$_{12}$–dependent enzyme identified thus far in man is the coenzyme B$_{12}$–dependent methylmalonyl-CoA mutase. This enzyme has been isolated from animal tissue and found to have a molecular weight of 165,000, and two moles of cobalt per mole of enzyme. The holoenzyme is stable, but the apoenzyme is unstable. The enzyme functions in the conversion of L-methylmalonyl-CoA to succinyl-CoA by facilitating an intramolecular and probably an intermolecular transfer of hydrogen on the L-methylmalonyl-CoA molecule to form succinyl-CoA. Decreased activity of this enzyme in pernicious anemia is believed to account for the production of increased amounts of metabolites proximal to methylmalonyl-CoA, such as propionate, and to account for the conversion of methylmalonyl-CoA into methylmalonic acid that appears in the urine of patients with pernicious anemia.

CHAPTER 8

INTRINSIC FACTOR

From the earliest description of Combe[96] in 1822, in which the possibility was raised that a disorder of the "digestive tract" could be a causative factor of the anemia, various investigators over a span of more than a century became increasingly aware that certain disorders of the stomach had an important etiological relationship to pernicious anemia. The observations of Flint,[149] Cahn and von Mering,[67] Levine and Ladd,[273] and Hurst[221] demonstrate the evolution of this concept starting with a suggestion by Flint in 1860[149] and culminating in the firm recognition by Levine and Ladd[273] and by Hurst[221] that achlorhydria was a *sine qua non* for the confident diagnosis of pernicious anemia.

William B. Castle[78,79] was aware of these historical precedents regarding the stomach and pernicious anemia. In a series of remarkably pragmatic and ingenious studies beginning in 1927,[78-83] and utilizing "such kitchen type equipment as a meat chopper, yellow bowl, spoon, and strainer,... and the essential analyzer: the patient,"* he and his colleagues elucidated the physiological and physiochemical basis of the gastric abnormalities in pernicious anemia. As a result of these studies, and for the first time in the history of the evolution of knowledge of pernicious anemia, Castle et al. advanced an acceptable theory based on sound experimental evidence regarding the etiology of this disorder. Extensive reviews regarding the isolation and properties of Castle's intrinsic factor have subsequently been published.[84-86,164,202]

---

*W. B. Castle, personal communication to the author.

ORIGIN OF INTRINSIC FACTOR

Following Glass et al.'s report[162] that intrinsic factor was a "glandular mucoprotein," Hoedemaeker et al.[213] determined by autoradiographic techniques that intrinsic factor was produced in the parietal cells of human stomach and in the chief cells of the rat stomach. Using an immunofluorescence technique and autoantibodies, Fisher and Taylor[148] confirmed Hoedemaeker et al.'s observations by reporting that some pernicious anemia sera contained antibodies against an intrinsic factor antigen that was present in gastric parietal cells.

PROPERTIES OF INTRINSIC FACTOR

Intrinsic factor has proved to be an elusive substance, and numerous attempts have been made to isolate and purify it. Although it has not been obtained in pure form as yet, certain properties of partially purified intrinsic factor have been delineated.[103,164,176] To date it is known that intrinsic factor is:

1. A glycoprotein with molecular weight of approximately 50,000-60,000. Higher molecular weight dimers may form in the presence of vitamin B_{12}.

2. Composed of two components that have been called S and I.[175,176]

3. Thermosensitive, especially in the case of intrinsic factor from human stomach. Intrinsic factor in extracted human gastric mucosa is less thermolabile at alkaline pH.

4. Nondialyzable and nonultrafiltrable, but filtrable through a Berkefield filter.

5. Relatively resistant to storage and freeze-drying at neutral pH, but it undergoes slow and progressive loss of activity at low pH.

6. Resistant to alkaline pH up to 10. Above pH 11.5, there is loss of intrinsic factor activity. At pH 12.6, intrinsic factor dissociates from the intrinsic factor–vitamin B_{12} complex.[176]

7. Slowly and partially inactivated by pepsin and resistant to digestion by trypsin and papain.

8. Seemingly "protected" from digestion by pepsin and chymotrypsin if it is bound to vitamin B_{12} in an intrinsic factor–vitamin B_{12} complex.

9. Precipitable by ammonium sulfate at 46% to 55% saturation, cold ethanol at 70% to 95% saturation, and cold acetone at 40% to 80% saturation. The latter two precipitates demonstrate some loss of intrinsic factor activity.

10. Devoid of blood group activity.[103] Any blood group substance activity that is detected is generally considered to be a contaminant or a complex of mucopolysaccharides and intrinsic factor.

11. Highly specific in terms of its vitamin B_{12} binding ability. The vitamin B_{12} binding sites on the intrinsic factor molecule contain tyrosine,[176] and these sites have a stereochemical preference for the cobalamin structure.[63,172]

12. Believed to undergo a "contraction" or "shrinking" of its molecular radius after binding to vitamin B_{12}.[176]

BINDING OF INTRINSIC FACTOR TO VITAMIN B_{12}

Aside from the small amounts (approximately 1%) of vitamin B_{12} that are absorbed passively throughout the small intestine by diffusion,[203] the initial essential step in the absorption of the majority of the vitamin is its attachment to intrinsic factor. A number of investigators have studied factors involved in the binding of intrinsic factor to vitamin B_{12}.[2,13,47,209,264,285,363] Gräsbeck et al.[175,176] found that there were two components in human gastric juice that possessed intrinsic factor activity. These were called S and I and were prepared as their cyanocobalamin complexes. The former was homogeneous and the latter was a more purified form. The complex had an S=m60 of 115,111 and had two moles of cobalamin per mole and 13% carbohydrate. Complex I was small and was a degradation product of S, the original intrinsic factor. Both complexes were regarded as polymers and probably dimers. A third vitamin B_{12} binder in gastric juice has been called R binder[176] and is said to be immunologically distinct from intrinsic factor. It has a molecular weight of approximately 110,000 and may be closely related to or the same as transcobalamin I.[176]

Schade et al.[363] determined that there might be more than one binding site for vitamin B_{12} on the intrinsic factor molecule. They reported that the antibody activity that blocked the binding of vitamin B_{12} by intrinsic factor (Antibody I) was on a molecule different from that which reacted with the intrinsic factor–vitamin B_{12} complex. The authors interpreted their results as indicating that intrinsic factor had at least two antigenic regions capable of binding vitamin B_{12}. Bunge and Schilling[63] found that vitamin B_{12} analogues competed for the binding sites on the intrinsic factor molecule but that gastric juice seemed preferentially to bind cyanocobalamin. They noted that the majority of the vitamin B_{12} molecule was bound by gastric juice and did not dissociate from the gastric juice in the presence of added excess vitamin B_{12} molecules.

The specificity of the intrinsic factor–vitamin B_{12} binding was investigated by Gottlieb et al.[172] who found that all vitamin B_{12}-like substances tested except 5,6-dimethylbenzimidazole and cobaloxime bound well to nonintrinsic factor vitamin B_{12} binders. Conversely, only intrinsic factor antibodies and cyanocobalamin blocked radioactive B_{12} binding to intrinsic factor. Vitamin B_{12} binders in pernicious anemia gastric juice were not effectively blocked by either intrinsic factor antibody or analogues.

McGuigan[285] measured the affinity of vitamin B_{12} for intrinsic factor using an equilibrium dialysis technique that included antisera inhibition of intrinsic factor binding of vitamin B_{12}. He found that intrinsic factor had a marked affinity for vitamin B_{12} $(0.38 \pm 0.07) \times 10^{10}$ M^{-1}. The strength of the binding in the intrinsic factor–B_{12} complex was not dependent on the hydrogen ion concentration. The intrinsic factor–B_{12} complex is susceptible to digestion by pronase.[314] Abels and Schilling[2] determined that vitamin B_{12} "protected" intrinsic factor, since the intrinsic factor–vitamin B_{12} complex was less vulnerable to autogenous digestion and heat than intrinsic factor alone. The authors speculated that achlorhydria was an important defense mechanism in the preservation of existing intrinsic factor in patients with pernicious anemia.

This protection of the intrinsic factor–vitamin B_{12} complex from autogenous digestion is also believed to result in part from a unique stereoconfiguration of the intrinsic factor–B_{12} complex itself.[176,362] Gräsbeck[176] has postulated that the nucleotide portion of the vitamin B_{12} molecule fits into a "pit" on the surface of the intrinsic factor molecule, and the cyanide side of the corrin plane faces outward from the molecule. The entry of the nucleotide portion of the cyanocobalamin molecule into the "pit" of the intrinsic factor molecule is said to cause a conformational change in the intrinsic factor molecule described as a "shrinking" or "contraction." This shrinking, according to measurements performed by Gräsbeck, leads to a molecular complex of intrinsic factor and vitamin B_{12} that is stereochemically more spherical than intrinsic factor alone, and more resistant to autogenous digestion than vitamin B_{12} alone, since the nucleotide portion of the vitamin is "protected" within the "pit" of the intrinsic factor molecule.

INTRINSIC FACTOR ASSAYS

The original intrinsic factor assays were bioassays, dependent upon untreated pernicious anemia patients and developed by Castle et al.[78-82] In view of this, Minot and Castle[299] discussed the interpretation of the reticulocyte reactions and their value in assessing the potency of intrinsic factor preparations. Ellenbogen and Williams[137] subsequently described a quantitative bioassay of intrinsic factor activity using the urinary excretion of radioactive vitamin B_{12}.

Recently, Sullivan et al.[389] developed an *in vitro* assay for human intrinsic factor. They used a homogenate from the distal half of a guinea pig small intestine in their assay system. Antibodies to human stomach mucosa inhibited the uptake of vitamin B_{12} mediated by human gastric juice in their experiments. Intrinsic factor was found to be heat labile, labile below pH 3.5, and moderately stable to alkaline pH. It was inhibited by acidity of intestinal milieu *in vivo* and *in vitro*. The activity of gastric juice in the homogenates was reversibly decreased at pH 5.8 and below, destroyed by heat or prolonged exposure to acid, and not destroyed by moderately alkaline pH or by storage at $-20°C$ at neutral pH.

The assay of intrinsic factor in various disorders of the stomach other than atrophic gastritis has also been performed. Goldhamer[168] found that pernicious anemia could develop in patients with carcinoma of the stomach, presumably as a result of failure of production of intrinsic factor by the neoplasm. Ardeman and Chanarin[16] found that the concentration of intrinsic factor in the gastric juice of patients with partial gastrectomy was decreased and similar to that found in patients with pernicious anemia.

The variability of intrinsic factor secretion in patients with pernicious anemia has been reported by several authors,[82,167] and intrinsic factor can be detected in the gastric juice in the absence of any stimulant to gastric secretion.[12] Inadequate intrinsic factor output per day is believed to result from inadequate secretion of gastric juice containing a normal concentration of intrinsic factor, from secretion of a normal volume of gastric juice with a decreased concentration of intrinsic factor, or from a combination of these factors.

SUMMARY

Intrinsic factor is a glycoprotein of high molecular weight produced by the parietal cells of the gastric mucosa. It is thermosensitive, nondialyzable and nonultrafiltrable, relatively resistant to freeze-drying and neutral pH and to storage, susceptible to loss of activity especially at low pH, resistant to alkaline pH up to 10, and susceptible to decrease in activity at pH greater than 11.5. Intrinsic factor is slowly and partially inactivated by pepsin, but this loss of activity is mitigated when the intrinsic factor is bound to vitamin B_{12}. The preservation of intrinsic factor activity when exposed to trypsin and papain is also improved if the intrinsic factor is bound to vitamin B_{12}.

Intrinsic factor is precipitable by cold ethanol at 70% to 95% saturation, ammonium sulfate at 46% to 55% saturation, and cold acetone at 40% to 80% saturation. Intrinsic factor preparations may possess blood group substance activity that may be presumed to be either a contaminant or a feature of mucopolysaccharides that can form a complex with intrinsic factor.

There are at least two components in human gastric juice identified thus far that possess intrinsic factor activity, and there may be more than one binding site for vitamin B_{12} on the intrinsic factor molecule. Of the various vitamin B_{12} analogues, cyanocobalamin binds most avidly to intrinsic factor. The affinity of vitamin B_{12} for intrinsic factor is high, and the strength of the binding is not dependent upon hydrogen ion concentration. It is believed by some that vitamin B_{12} protects intrinsic factor against autogenous digestion. One mechanism that has been proposed for this protective action is that the nucleotide portion of the vitamin B_{12} moiety fits into a pit on the surface of the intrinsic factor molecule, causing a conformational change in the form of shrinkage or contraction of the molecule.

In vivo assays for intrinsic factor have been known since the early descriptions of this substance by Castle. Newer *in vitro* techniques utilizing intestinal homogenates and antibodies to human gastric mucosa have also been described. The secretion of intrinsic factor may be variable in patients with pernicious anemia, and inadequate intrinsic factor secretion may be the result of several interrelating factors.

CHAPTER 9

AUTOIMMUNITY
IN PERNICIOUS ANEMIA

Antibodies to both parietal cells and to intrinsic factor are found in the gastrointestinal tract and sera of most patients with pernicious anemia.[74,227] To date, however, the role of these antibodies in the pathogenesis of atrophic gastritis and the development of intrinsic factor deficiency is uncertain.[205,223]

A number of early studies using known immunosuppressive agents such as corticosteroids suggested the possibilities of autoimmune factors in pernicious anemia. Thorn et al.[401] mentioned that in a case of Gardner, who treated a 52-year-old woman with pernicious anemia with ACTH for five days, increased reticulocytes (to 7.5%) were seen, followed by a decline in the reticulocyte count. The reticulocytosis was accompanied by an increase in nucleated red cells (up to 52%). There was no significant increase in the red blood cell count, but the bone marrow was said to show a "marked change in the red cell series from a very immature to a mature type of cell." This picture reverted to pretreatment status nine days after cessation of ACTH therapy.

Wintrobe et al.[439] treated two patients with pernicious anemia with ACTH. No symptomatic improvement was noted, but a slight increase in reticulocytes without change in hematocrit or mean corpuscular volume occurred. Doig et al.[118] reported an unexpected hematopoietic response to prednisolone in a patient with rheumatoid arthritis who also had pernicious anemia. In eight patients treated with steroids, there was conversion of megaloblastic to normoblastic erythropoiesis. However, the authors did not recommend prednisolone therapy for pernicious anemia.

Following the clinical observations that steroids could lead to hematological improvement in pernicious anemia, various investigators reported the presence of antibodies to intrinsic factor in the serum and gastric juice of patients with pernicious anemia. Most of the available evidence to date supports the postulate that there are two types of antibodies to intrinsic factor: one is a blocking antibody that blocks the binding of intrinsic factor to vitamin B_{12}, and the second is a binding (precipitating) antibody that combines with the intrinsic factor–vitamin B_{12} complex.

Serum antibodies to intrinsic factor were first detected by Schwartz,[368] and his report was also the first to indicate that autoimmune phenomena may occur in pernicious anemia. In certain patients with pernicious anemia treated with an oral vitamin B_{12}–intrinsic factor preparation, Schwartz noted the development of what seemed to be an acquired resistance to intrinsic factor. In the serum of some of these patients he detected inhibitors to intrinsic factor, although these inhibitors were not found in the sera of untreated pernicious anemia patients. Subsequently, Taylor[393] demonstrated that intrinsic factor activity could be inhibited by the serum of both treated and untreated pernicious anemia patients. In three patients hydrocortisone decreased the inhibitory effect but the capacity to absorb vitamin B_{12} was not increased. Taylor concluded that the inhibitory factor may be a true antibody and perhaps an autoantibody.

Saliva and gastric juice of patients with pernicious anemia may also contain antibodies to intrinsic factor. Carmel and Herbert[76] found precipitating antibody against intrinsic factor in the saliva of patients with pernicious anemia. The antibody was IgA, and it could neutralize intrinsic factor activity. The authors postulated that the intrinsic factor antibody in saliva could aggravate vitamin B_{12} deficiency. Carmel and Herbert[74] also determined that the blocking type of antibody to intrinsic factor was more frequently found in the ileum, whereas the precipitating antibody was more frequent in gastric juice. At least one of the two antibodies was postulated to be positive in nearly all patients with pernicious anemia.

Fisher et al.[147] also detected an inhibitor to intrinsic factor in the gastric juice of patients with pernicious anemia and found that it was an autoantibody specific for intrinsic factor. Schade et al.[362] reported the case of a 72-year-old man with megaloblastic anemia, achlorhydria, and antibodies to intrinsic factor in his serum. The patient did not absorb vitamin B_{12} from a mixture of normal gastric juice or vitamin B_{12} given orally. His gastric juice contained antibodies to a complex of human intrinsic factor and vitamin B_{12}. This antibody led to decreased absorption of vitamin B_{12}. In contrast to the studies of others, Yates and Cooper[443] did not find intrinsic factor antibodies in the gastrointestinal secretions of seven patients with pernicious anemia, and therefore could not implicate antibodies in the pathogenesis of vitamin B_{12} malabsorption.

Studies utilizing porcine intrinsic factor have also contributed to the understanding of intrinsic factor antibodies in pernicious anemia. Kaplan et al.[237] studied two patients with pernicious anemia who were injected with purified hog intrinsic factor until they developed sensitivity. However, refractoriness to oral hog intrinsic factor did not occur. They postulated that in patients refractory to intrinsic factor the refractoriness occurred because of local factors in the gastrointestinal tract. Ardeman and Chanarin[14] found that hog intrinsic factor had a greater ability to absorb vitamin B_{12} than human intrinsic factor because the villi of human intestine contained an antibody to human intrinsic factor.

The relationship between blood group substances and intrinsic factor antibodies was studied by Samloff et al.[360] They reported that the incidence of intrinsic factor binding antibodies was greater in patients with blood group O than with group A. The concentration of blocking antibodies was higher in sera that also contained binding antibodies than in sera with only blocking antibodies.

Recent experiments by Tai and McGuigan[391] have indicated that immunologically competent cells may participate in the pathogenesis of intrinsic factor antibodies. These authors studied peripheral blood lymphocyte-rich leukocyte preparations from 29 patients with pernicious anemia cultured in the presence of gastric juice or intrinsic factor. Lymphocyte transformation was exhibited in only those patients whose sera did not contain blocking antibodies to the intrinsic factor.

The results of their study are consistent with the interpretation that the peripheral blood lymphocytes (immunocytes) in patients with pernicious anemia may be capable of responding immunologically to an antigenic challenge with intrinsic factor. Their report also suggests that the serum and gastric autoantibodies to intrinsic factor may have a basis in cellular as well as humoral immunity. The finding of intrinsic factor antibodies within the cytoplasm of plasma cells in the bone marrow of patients with pernicious anemia (Chapter 10) is further evidence of the role of immunologically competent cells in the pathogenesis of these antibodies.

An additional demonstration of the presence of cellular immunity in the pathogenesis of antibodies to intrinsic factor was provided by Baur et al.[28] They found that in gastric biopsies from patients with pernicious anemia, mononuclear inflammatory cells contained antibodies against intrinsic factor. Presumably, these antibodies were produced by the inflammatory cells.

Antibodies to parietal cells may also be found in the serum and gastric juice of patients with pernicious anemia. These antibodies, as well as the antibodies to intrinsic factor, are believed to be produced by mononuclear inflammatory cells within the gastric mucosa[28] and in plasma cells in the bone marrow of patients with pernicious anemia

(Chapter 10). In contrast to intrinsic factor antibodies, the incidence of parietal cell antibodies was found to be independent of blood group substances,[360] and there did not appear to be a correlation between the presence or absence of lymphocyte transformation and the presence or absence of serum antibodies to parietal cells.[391]

The occurrence of parietal cell antibodies in pernicious anemia has been studied by several authors. Jeffries and Sleisenger[227] found gastric parietal cell antibodies by immunofluorescence in sera from 62 of 72 patients with pernicious anemia. The parietal cell antibody was present in the IgA fraction and was also found in gastric juice from pernicious anemia patients. Parietal cell antibody was not found in mucosal extracts.

Antibodies to parietal cells are not found exclusively in patients with pernicious anemia, as is the case with intrinsic factor antibodies. Adams et al.[5] found that in 20 patients with gastric parietal antibodies in the serum without pernicious anemia, the parietal cell autoantibodies in the serum were associated with chronic gastritis. In Fisher's and Taylor's study,[146] 85% of the patients with pernicious anemia had parietal cell antibodies detectable by immunofluorescence. Of their patients with chronic gastritis, 62.5% had parietal cell antibodies, but none of the patients with chronic gastritis had antibodies to intrinsic factor.

These studies support the viewpoint that although antibodies to parietal cells may be found in a large number of patients with pernicious anemia, they are not specific for this disorder since they may occur in a substantial percentage of patients with chronic gastritis. In addition, the mechanisms of cellular immunity in the pathogenesis of antibodies to parietal cells may differ from those seen in the case of intrinsic factor antibodies.[391] Not all of the secretory capacities of gastric epithelial cells are affected in the atrophic gastritis found in pernicious anemia. Serum gastrin levels measured by immunoassay are unusually high in this disorder,[188] reflecting the ability of the gastrin secreting cells in an otherwise atrophic gastritis to elaborate gastrin in response to acid and secretin stimuli.

Additional studies have demonstrated that treatment of pernicious anemia with corticosteroids may increase both intrinsic factor secretion and hydrochloric acid output. The results of these studies have been interpreted as constituting additional evidence for the pathogenetic role of autoimmune substances in pernicious anemia, since immunosuppressive agents such as corticosteroids led to improvement in those parameters believed to be affected by these autoantibodies.

An increase in activity of intrinsic factor after treatment of pernicious anemia by corticosteroids was found by Kristensen and Friis.[255] These authors suggested that prednisone could stimulate the production of intrinsic factor in patients with pernicious anemia.

Ardeman and Chanarin[15] found that in some patients with pernicious anemia treated with prednisolone, a return of hydrochloric acid and intrinsic factor to the gastric juice and return of chief and parietal cells to the gastric mucosa were observed. In some of these patients, improvement in vitamin B_{12} absorption also occurred, but a demonstrable increase in intrinsic factor was not found in all patients. Improvement took place both in patients with intrinsic factor antibodies and in those without intrinsic factor antibodies in the serum. Steroids had no effect on the absorption of vitamin B_{12} in patients who had partial or total gastrectomies.

Jeffries et al.[228] also noted that after treatment of five pernicious anemia patients with prednisolone, gastric glands containing parietal and chief cells reappeared in the mucosal biopsies during steroid therapy. The reappearance of parietal cells was associated with return of acid secretion in three patients and with return of intrinsic factor secretion in each of the five patients. Serum titers of parietal cell antibodies were unchanged, but there was a decrease in intrinsic factor antibody titer in two patients. In all of the patients with pernicious anemia, prednisolone therapy enhanced the absorption of vitamin B_{12}.

SUMMARY

In the serum and gastric juice of the majority of patients with pernicious anemia, antibodies to intrinsic factor and to parietal cells may be found. Two kinds of antibody to intrinsic factor have been characterized. These are the blocking and the precipitating antibodies. Blocking antibody against intrinsic factor is found more frequently in the ileum, and precipitating antibody is detected more often in the gastric juice. Precipitating antibody against intrinsic factor is also found in the saliva of patients with pernicious anemia and has been identified as an IgA globulin. Antibodies against parietal cells may be found in patients who have chronic gastritis, whereas intrinsic factor antibodies are usually not detectable in these patients. Parietal cell antibodies have been reported to be directed against a microsomal component of gastric parietal cells.

Apparent remissions of pernicious anemia after the administration of corticosteroids are believed to result in part from suppression of immune reactions that are responsible for the production of these antibodies and consequent aggravation of the vitamin B_{12} deficiency. In some patients with pernicious anemia treated with corticosteroids, it has been reported that hydrochloric acid and intrinsic factor reappeared in the gastric juice.

The role of autoantibodies in the pathogenesis of pernicious anemia is uncertain. The studies of Tai and McGuigan[391] suggest that immunologically competent cells (lymphocytes) may be involved in the autoimmune phenomena insofar as intrinsic factor antibodies are concerned. Although antibodies to both parietal cells and intrinsic factor may be present in the ileum and gastric juice of most patients with pernicious anemia, to date it is not generally accepted that pernicious anemia is *per se* an autoimmune disorder (Chapter 10).

RELATIONSHIPS BETWEEN PERNICIOUS ANEMIA AND MYXEDEMA

A number of investigators have reported that the incidence of pernicious anemia is increased in patients with idiopathic primary myxedema, and they have speculated that both pernicious anemia and myxedema may have a basis in autoimmunity. Charcot[91] in 1881 mentioned that anemia occurred in some patients with myxedema, although the nature of this anemia was not defined. Putnam[335] also reported the occurrence of anemia in some patients with myxedema. Bramwell[57] stated that in myxedema, "some anemia is usually present... but the alterations in the blood do not present any notable peculiarities."

Minot[296] in 1921 was among the first to provide a detailed description of the blood in myxedema. In his Case 2 of "Two curable cases of anemia," Minot observed in a case of myxedema with anemia that the erythrocytes were "a trifle oval," but large macrocytes were not seen. Minot remarked that in rare cases the erythrocytes in myxedema could resemble those seen in pernicious anemia. Emery[138] found that eight of fourteen patients with myxedema had anemia, but the blood picture was inconstant. There was no mention of macrocytosis, and Emery stated that the anemia disappeared after treatment of the hypothyroidism.

Lerman and Means[270] were the first to systematically study gastric secretions in patients with Graves' disease and myxedema. They found that in patients with either disorder, gastric acidity was approximately 50% of normal. Achlorhydria in Graves' disease had an incidence of 38%, and in myxedema the incidence was 53%. The authors noted that patients who had myxedema and achlorhydria had an "unusual tendency" to develop anemia.

According to Sturgis,[387] approximately 50% of patients with myxedema have achlorhydria. At the Simpson Memorial Institute, patients who had myxedema and achlorhydria often had macrocytic anemias that were treated elsewhere with liver extract. Because they did not show a hematological response, they were believed to have "refractory pernicious anemia." Subsequently it was found that the achlorhydria in these patients disappeared after treatment of the myxedema with thyroid, and the anemia also remitted. Apparently, both the achlorhydria and anemia were related to hypothyroidism in these patients.

Tudhope and Wilson[405] also studied the anemia of hypothyroidism. In 166 cases of hypothyroidism, mild nonspecific anemia was found in 5 patients. In 13 patients (7.8%) true pernicious anemia was found. In their studies, macrocytic anemia in hypothyroidism apart from pernicious anemia was rare. In a subsequent study, Tudhope and Wilson[406] studied vitamin B_{12} deficiency in hypothyroidism. They found that of 73 patients with primary spontaneous hypothyroidism, 24 of 52 patients tested had achlorhydria. Of the 73 patients, 9 had pernicious anemia, and of 52 patients tested, 7 had vitamin B_{12} deficiency without pernicious anemia.

In summary, macrocytic anemia occurring in idiopathic primary myxedema is usually related to the hypothyroidism and ordinarily improves after the administration of thyroid hormone. In some patients with myxedema, achlorhydria may also occur. If such patients are also anemic, they may be suspected of having pernicious anemia. However, both the achlorhydria and anemia may disappear after treatment with thyroid hormone. A group of patients with myxedema may also have achlorhydria that does not disappear after treatment of the hypothyroidism, and in some of these patients the macrocytic anemia may be true pernicious anemia. In addition, antithyroid antibodies may be detectable in the serum of certain pernicious anemia patients, although at the time these individuals may not be clinically hypothyroid.

The relationship of idiopathic myxedema to autoimmunity is uncertain, as is the relationship of pernicious anemia to autoimmunity. Nevertheless, there is a current belief that pernicious anemia, idiopathic myxedema, and Addison's disease (idiopathic hypoadrenalism) may all have an autoimmune etiology and that combinations of these disorders may occur in a single patient.

CHAPTER 10

PATHOGENETIC ASPECTS OF PERNICIOUS ANEMIA

PATHOGENESIS OF MEGALOBLASTIC ERYTHROPOIESIS

Approximately 19 years after the advent of panoptic stains[128] and their application to hematological diagnosis, Cabot[64] in 1898 wrote that

> The typical megaloblast is an abnormally large cell ... frequently showing marks of degeneration (polychromatophilia) in its protoplasm, which is therefore brownish or purplish with the Ehrlich-Biondi stain. Its nucleus is very large, filling most of the cell, and contrasts with the normoblast nucleus, not only by its greater size but by the pale, even stain which it takes up. The commonest color of the nucleus ... is pale green or robin's-egg color. It is not stained evenly but dotted over with purplish granules arranged in a fine mesh like the knots in a fish net.

A reproduction of megaloblasts from Cabot's 1898 textbook[64] is illustrated in Figure 99. Ehrlich and Lazarus[133] in 1905 also described the nucleus of the megaloblast in pernicious anemia as having "much less marked affinity" for the usual nuclear stains available at the time. Reproductions of megaloblasts from Lazarus' chapter in Nothnagel's 1905 textbook[265] are shown in Figure 100. Cabot's[64] and Ehrlich's and Lazarus'[133] remarkable insights based on rudimentary techniques of staining and microscopy by modern-day standards may be considered among the earliest observations that there was something unique about the nuclear chromatin of the megaloblast in pernicious anemia.

Why megaloblastic nuclear chromatin is finely attenuated, why there are few chromatin aggregates in well-developed megaloblasts, why the chromatin strands are widely separated, imparting a fenestrated appearance to the nucleus, are all challenging and as yet unanswered questions in the area of nucleoprotein biochemistry in per-

186

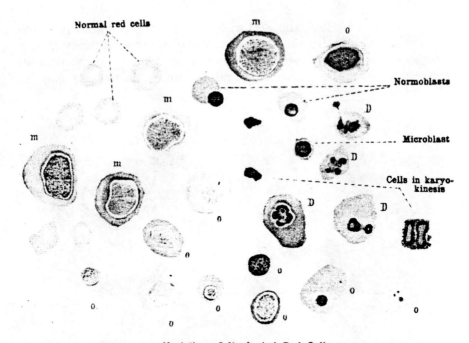

Normal red cells

m

0

Normoblasts

m

D

Microblast

m

D

m

Cells in karyo-
kinesis

D

D

0

0

0

0

0

0

0

0

0

0

0

Varieties of Nucleated Red Cells.
m. m. m. m. = Typical megaloblasts.   D. D. D. D. = Cells with dividing nuclei.
o. o. o. o. o. o. o. = Other (unnamed) varieties of nucleated red corpuscles.

Figure 99. Megaloblasts (labeled "m") in the peripheral blood of a patient with pernicious anemia, as illustrated by Cabot in 1898. (From Cabot, R. C. *A Guide to the Clinical Examination of the Blood for Diagnostic Purposes.* W. Wood & Co., New York, 1898, p. 93.)

nicious anemia. Indeed, why the megaloblast is a megaloblast at all—that is, why a deficiency of a vitamin should cause a cell to enlarge—is still one of the fundamental unanswered questions in pernicious anemia and in the anemia of folate deficiency.

Figure 100. Megaloblasts (labeled "a") as illustrated by Lazarus in 1905. (From Lazarus, A. Progressive Pernicious Anemia, in Stengel, A. (ed.) *Diseases of the Blood,* W. B. Saunders, Philadelphia, 1905, p. 254. Reproduced with permission of W. B. Saunders Co.)

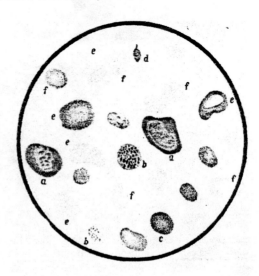

Although megaloblastic erythropoiesis is usually found in nutritional (i.e., vitamin B_{12} or folate deficient) anemias, at times it may occur in erythroid disorders that are not associated with demonstrable deficiencies of these vitamins. Megaloblastic erythropoiesis may be

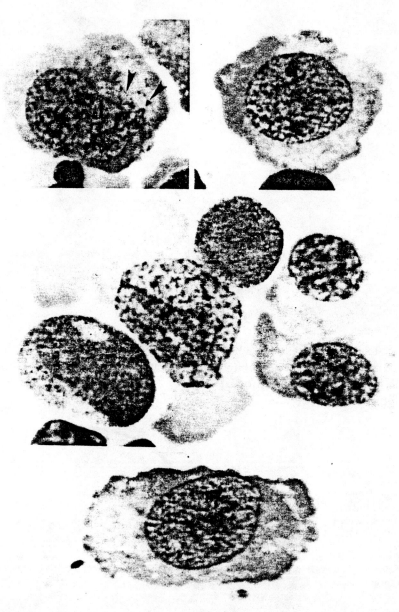

Figure 101. Giant intermediate megaloblasts from the bone marrow of a patient with erythroleukemia who had normal serum vitamin B_{12} and folate levels. The nuclear chromatin is exceptionally attenuated and chromatin aggregates are seen rarely. Nucleocytoplasmic asynchrony is present. Arrows point to a Cabot ring in the cytoplasm of one of the erythroid precursors (top, left).

seen rarely in pyridoxine-responsive sideroblastic anemia and on occasion may be found in erythroleukemia. Examples of unusually severe megaloblastic changes in erythroid precursors from a patient with erythroleukemia are seen in Figure 101. To date, the pathogenesis of megaloblastosis in erythroleukemia and in certain rare cases of pyridoxine-responsive sideroblastic anemias is unknown, but it may reflect an inability of erythroid precursors in these disorders to properly utilize vitamin B_{12} or folate, or both.

In visualizing the pathological changes in erythroid precursors in pernicious anemia, it appears as though with increasing severity of the anemia there is progressive attenuation or thinning of chromatin strands and corresponding loss of chromatin aggregates. A normal intermediate normoblast is shown in Figure 102. Large aggregates of chromatin are connected to each other by coarse-appearing chromatin strands. In erythroid precursors obtained from patients with minimal pernicious anemia, areas of focal attenuation of chromatin strands can be observed (Fig. 103). At times these thinned chromatin strands seem to be localized in one area of the nucleus. In other instances, the attenuated areas are scattered throughout the nucleus. A "clockface"

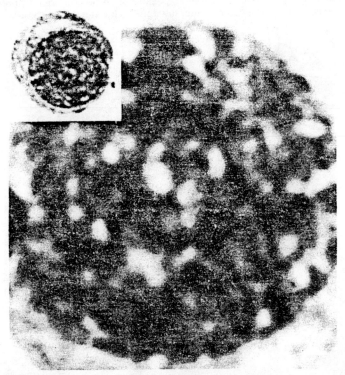

Figure 102. Normal intermediate normoblast (inset), and higher power view of nuclear chromatin. There are numerous large aggregates of chromatin, and coarse, ropelike connections between the aggregates.

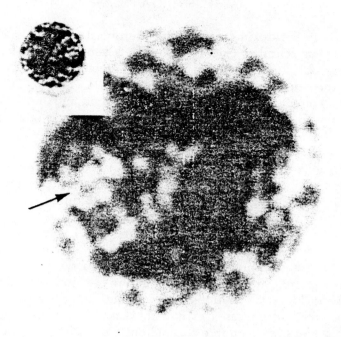

Figure 103. Intermediate megaloblast from patient with minimal pernicious anemia (inset). The higher power view of the nucleus shows areas where there is focal attenuation of chromatin strands (arrow). Large aggregates of chromatin are still present. The chromatin adjacent to the nuclear membrane appears attenuated and sparse.

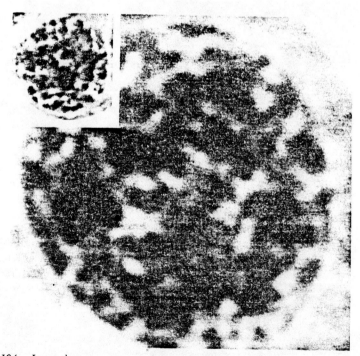

Figure 104. Inset shows an intermediate megaloblast from a patient with mild pernicious anemia. In the higher power view, blocklike aggregates of chromatin are present, but the connections between them appear attenuated and the nucleus has acquired a fenestrated appearance.

190

chromatin pattern[238] exhibiting isolated "hillocks" and "clumps" of chromatin surrounding the inner circumference of the nuclear membrane may be seen.

As the anemia becomes more severe, as seen in Figure 104, megaloblastic changes become more pronounced. Additional attenuated strands of chromatin are seen, and fewer aggregates of chromatin are found than in the earliest recognizable megaloblastic precursors illustrated in Figure 103.

Further worsening of the anemia is usually associated with additional thinning of the chromatin strands (Fig. 105), and at this point the chromatin strands begin to appear more widely separated, perhaps in part because they have become thinner. Aggregates of chromatin are less numerous than in the preceding type of megaloblastic precursors seen in Figures 103 and 104.

In the most severe cases of pernicious anemia, megaloblastic changes are the most pronounced as illustrated in Figure 106. The chromatin strands have become delicate-appearing and thread-like and often appear disconnected from other chromatin strands. In part

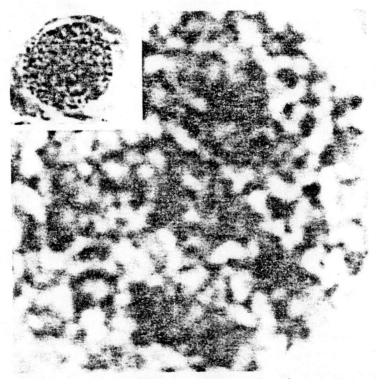

Figure 105. Intermediate megaloblast from a patient with moderate pernicious anemia (inset). The higher magnification of this cell shows that the number of chromatin aggregates is decreased, and the aggregates are smaller in size than those seen in Figures 103 and 104. The connections between chromatin aggregates are attenuated and delicate-appearing, and the nucleus appears fenestrated.

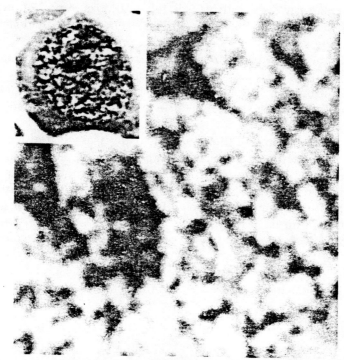

Figure 106. Inset shows a large intermediate megaloblast from a patient with severe pernicious anemia. In the higher power view, there are several aggregates of chromatin, but the majority of the nucleus is composed of delicate, interconnecting strands of chromatin. The few aggregates of chromatin are smaller than those in Figure 105 and have a knoblike appearance.

because of delicacy of the chromatin strands and the apparent widening of the distance between them, the megaloblast at this point appears markedly fenestrated with considerable open space between chromatin strands. Aggregates of chromatin may be greatly reduced in number and in some megaloblasts may be virtually absent.

A number of studies bear on the pathogenesis of the morphological lesion that we call megaloblastic.[110,122,230-233,241] Some of these are cytochemical studies based on fixed, stained preparations of megaloblasts. Others are biochemical and ultrastructural studies of nucleic acids and nucleoproteins including histones. Although the final explanation is far from complete, it may be possible, on the basis of the available information to date, to propose a theory of the pathogenesis of megaloblastic erythropoiesis found in pernicious anemia.

In terms of nucleic acids, various authors have demonstrated that there is a defect in the synthesis of DNA in pernicious anemia[30-36,292,434,444] and that this defect can be corrected by administration of vitamin B_{12}[165,398,436] and in some cases by the administration of various precursors of DNA such as thymine.[380,410] Beck[30-36] proposed that deficiency of vitamin B_{12} led to what he termed *unbalanced growth* in certain bacteria with the production of filamentous forms. He suggested that a similar phenomenon might occur in the case of the nuclear chromatin of the vitamin B_{12}–deficient erythroid precursor in which unbalanced growth of DNA strands would cause them to become filamentous, such as those visualized in a megaloblast stained with the Feulgen reagent to demonstrate DNA (Fig. 107).

Although Beck's data for bacterial forms appears convincing, it is uncertain whether a similar process of unbalanced growth occurs in the DNA of human erythroid precursors in vitamin B_{12} deficiency. The chromosomes of pernicious anemia erythroid precursors have been found to be longer than normal chromosomes,[331] perhaps supporting Beck's hypothesis. Recently, it has become possible to extract DNA and DNP (deoxyribonucleoprotein) from erythroid precursors in pernicious anemia and to examine the macromolecular configuration of these nucleic acids and nucleoproteins under high intensity electron microscopy using newly developed metallic shadowing techniques. Examples of DNA strands obtained from pernicious anemia proerythroblasts and megaloblasts are shown in Figure 108A and 108B. The

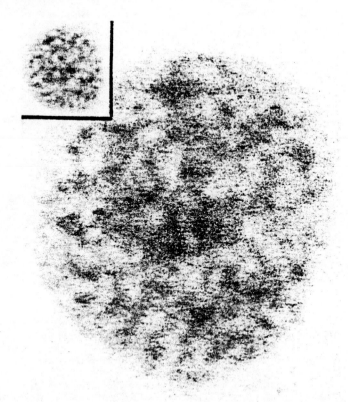

Figure 107. DNA in pernicious anemia megaloblast, demonstrated with the Feulgen stain. High power view of cell in the inset shows delicate-appearing strands of DNA and several small aggregates of DNA.

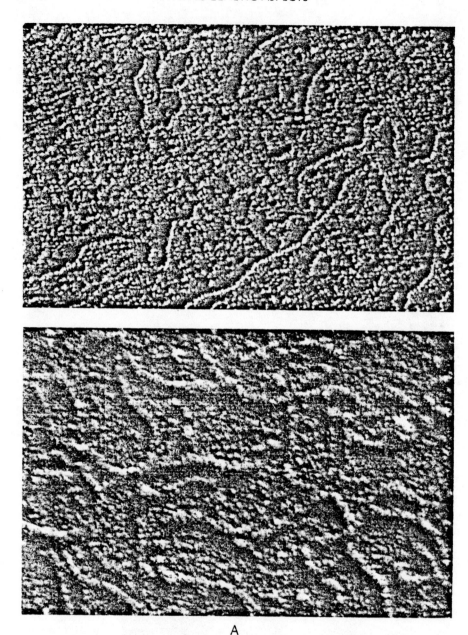

A

Figure 108. **A. Top:** the threadlike structures represented in this photograph are strands of highly purified DNA extracted primarily from proerythroblasts and early intermediate megaloblasts obtained from the bone marrow of a patient with severe untreated pernicious anemia. Films of a solution containing this DNA and cytochrome c were spread by the Kleinschmidt technique on 400-mesh copper grids coated with 100 Å thick carbon film and shadowed from a single direction with 80% platinum–20% palladium wire at a 10 degree angle. The grids were viewed with a JEM-6A transmission electron microscope operating at 80 KV accelerating voltage. (x 110,000 after enlargement.) **Bottom:** higher power view of strands of megaloblastic DNA obtained from a patient with severe untreated pernicious anemia. (x 260,000 after enlargement.) *Illustration continued on the opposite page.*

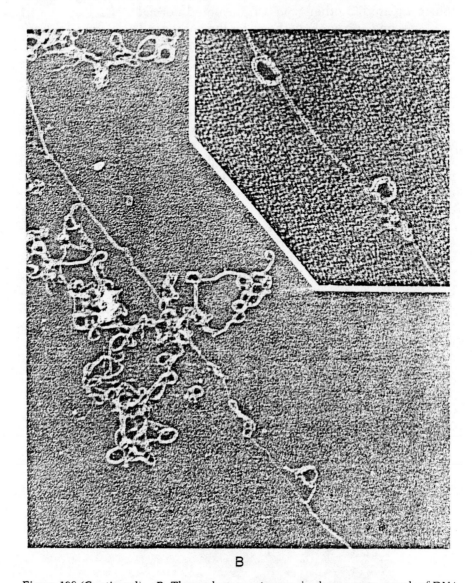

B

Figure 108 (Continued). **B.** These electron micrographs demonstrate strands of DNA extracted from the nuclei of pernicious anemia marrow cells, primarily proerythroblasts and megaloblasts. The DNA strands were spread on a carbon film activated by a 15 second exposure of the carbon to a 500 volt glow discharge in the presence of amylamine vapors. The electron micrographs were taken on a JEM-6A transmission electron microscope operating at 80 KV. The low power view at x 40,000 and the high power view (inset) at x 150,000 show double-stranded DNA apparently coiling to form thick strands in some areas and splitting into single strands in other places. This "activation" technique is believed to yield a more representative view of the macromolecular structure of the DNA strand than possible with the Kleinschmidt technique shown in *A*, since the DNA strands using the latter spreading process are coated with a layer of cytochrome c that is not present using the carbon activation method.

pernicious anemia DNA strands appear unusually thin and filamentous compared to other types of presumed normal DNA.

A second current hypothesis for the pathogenesis of megaloblastic erythropoiesis is the *methyltetrahydrofolate trap* concept.[49,61,62,201,206,229,292,312,313,396] This proposal states that in pernicious anemia there is a reduction in the activity of the methylcobalamin-dependent enzyme N^5-methyltetrahydrofolate-homocysteine methyltransferase.[396] Because of this block, N^5-methyltetrahydrofolate accumulates,[312] and there are reduced amounts of other folate intermediates such as tetrahydrofolate, dihydrofolate, and 5,10-methylenetetrahydrofolate available for the *de novo* synthesis of purines and pyrimidines. In particular, there is a deficiency of 5,10-methylenetetrahydrofolate, a substance that functions as a methyl donor in the methylation and subsequent conversion of deoxyuridine monophosphate to thymidine monophosphate.[253,292] The latter substance is a precursor of thymine DNA. Presumably, the defect in nucleic acid synthesis induced by the methyltetrahydrofolate trap leads to megaloblastosis. The methyltetrahydrofolate trap hypothesis states that the effects of vitamin B_{12} on the methylation of deoxyuridine monophosphate to thymidine monophosphate and ultimately to thymine DNA are mediated via folate and that a direct effect of vitamin B_{12} on nucleic acid synthesis has not as yet been demonstrated.

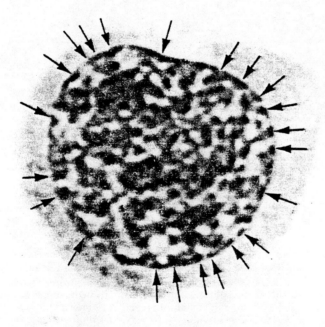

Figure 109.   Large intermediate megaloblast with typical fenestrated nuclear chromatin pattern and isolated clumps of chromatin adherent to the inner circumference of the nuclear membrane in a clockface pattern (arrows).

Histones, basic nucleoproteins that bind DNA together into compact masses of chromatin, have also been suggested as contributing to the pathogenesis of megaloblastic erythropoiesis in pernicious anemia.[238-242] The initial background for this postulate came about as the result of a morphological observation made in 1968.[238] An arrangement of nuclear chromatin surrounding the interior circumference of the nuclear membrane of megaloblasts in pernicious anemia was said to resemble a *clockface*. In this clockface chromatin pattern, which was found only in pernicious anemia and folate deficiency and not in other types of anemias, small isolated hillocks or clumps of nuclear chromatin were seen (Fig. 109).

It was proposed in this initial report[238] that the substance(s) responsible for binding chromatin together into compact masses and aggregates might be abnormal in pernicious anemia. Abnormalities of these binding substances (presumably histones) would contribute to the development of the seemingly isolated clumps and hillocks of nuclear chromatin, unconnected to other masses or strands of chromatin in megaloblasts. This clockface chromatin pattern has been observed in living megaloblasts viewed under phase contrast[3,42] as seen in Figure 110 and may also have an ultrastructural counterpart, as seen in an electron micrograph of an intermediate megaloblast in Figure 111. The dense heterochromatin of this cell appears to be in a circumferential arrangement around the interior of the nuclear membrane, similar to that seen in the light micrographs (Fig. 109). The

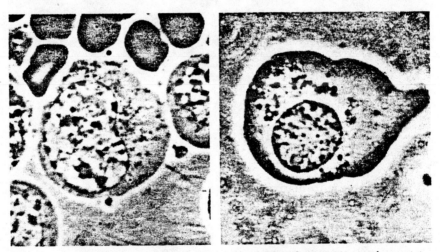

Figure 110. **Left:** large early intermediate megaloblast from patient with pernicious anemia, viewed under phase contrast. A clockface chromatin pattern is observed. (From Ackerman, A. and Bellios, N. C. Blood *10*:1183, 1955. Reproduced with permission of G. A. Ackerman, M.D., and Grune & Stratton, New York.) **Right:** late intermediate megaloblast from pernicious anemia patient, as viewed under phase contrast. Clumps of chromatin in a clockface pattern can be observed in this living megaloblast. (From Bessis, M. *Cytology of the Blood and Blood Forming Organs.* Grune & Stratton, New York, 1956. Reproduced with permission of Marcel Bessis, M.D., and Grune & Stratton, New York.)

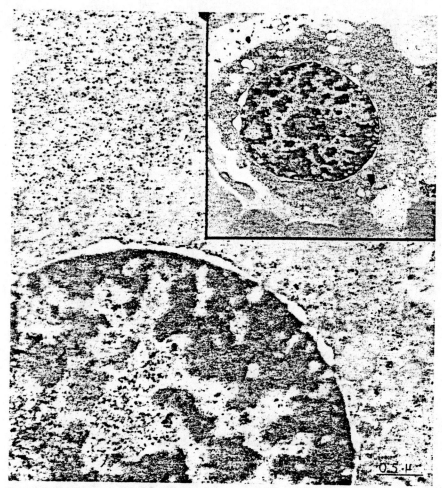

Figure 111. Electron micrograph of intermediate megaloblast (inset). As seen in the higher power view, seemingly isolated clumps of heterochromatin adherent to the inner surface of the nuclear membrane may constitute ultrastructural evidence of the clockface chromatin pattern as observed in both living megaloblasts and fixed-stained megaloblasts. The dark punctate structures in the cytoplasm represent ferritin. (Inset, x 7500; higher power view x 30,000.)

clumps of heterochromatin appear relatively unconnected to other masses of heterochromatin.

The initial morphological observation of the clockface chromatin pattern in megaloblasts[238] served as an impetus for a subsequent cytochemical study concerning the type of histones in the nuclei of pernicious anemia cells. This study used the ammoniacal silver stain[239] to distinguish between arginine-rich and lysine-rich histone in the nuclei of proerythroblasts from pernicious anemia and various other types of anemia as well as normal controls. Pernicious anemia proerythroblasts showed an unusual preponderance of lysine-rich histone (Plate 2 and Fig. 112A), and their nuclei stained bright yellow, indicating this type of histone. Only scant amounts of arginine-rich

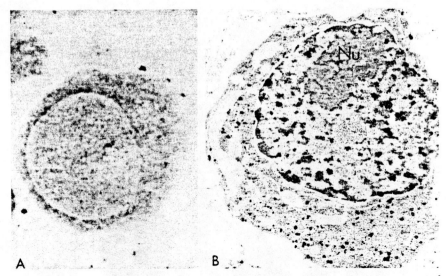

Figure 112. **A.** Proerythroblast or early intermediate megaloblast from a patient with severe pernicious anemia, stained with the ammoniacal silver stain to detect arginine-rich and lysine-rich histone. The nucleus stains homogeneously yellow, indicating predominantly lysine-rich histone, and dark punctate granules that would represent arginine-rich histone are observed rarely. **B.** Electron micrograph of pernicious anemia megaloblast fixed in acetate buffered formalin and stained with ammoniacal silver reagent, uranyl magnesium acetate, and lead citrate. Few dense black deposits representing sites of arginine-rich histones are localized in the heterochromatin of the nucleus. Occasional black granules appear in the cytoplasm as well and may represent sites of arginine-rich histone which is synthesized in the cytoplasm on polysomes. Nu = Nucleolus.

histone (black or brown punctate areas) were observed (Fig. 112A). Ultrastructurally, the ammoniacal silver reaction product is localized in the areas of heterochromatin as seen in Fig. 112B. Infrequent small deposits of silver representing sites of arginine-rich histone are seen in the heterochromatin, which is metabolically repressed inactive DNA.[245] In this initial cytochemical study the alkaline-fast green stain[239] also revealed a delicate network of histone threads and few small histone aggregates (Fig. 113).

With these cytochemical observations indicating abnormalities of histone in pernicious anemia, further biochemical studies were performed to elucidate the type(s) of abnormality. One study[240] examined the biosynthesis of arginine-rich histone in pernicious anemia megaloblasts before and after treatment with vitamin B_{12} *in vivo* and after exposure to coenzyme B_{12} *in vitro*. This study demonstrated a dramatic increase in the biosynthesis of arginine-rich histone after exposure to vitamin B_{12}. Autoradiographic evidence of uptake of ^3H arginine into the nuclei of megaloblasts is seen in Figure 114. Coincident with the marked uptake of tritium-labeled arginine into histone fractions extracted from the erythroid cells, there was a change in the electrophoretic pattern of the histones obtained before and after vitamin B_{12} exposure, as seen in Figure 115. These findings were interpreted as indicating that vitamin B_{12} could promote the biosynthesis of

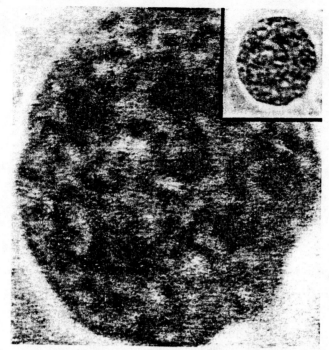

Figure 113. Megaloblast stained with alkaline-fast green to demonstrate histones (inset). The high power view of the nucleus shows a delicate network of histone threads and few small aggregates of histones that appear as "knobs" at junction points of histone strands.

arginine-rich histone in pernicious anemia megaloblasts and by doing so cause changes in the composition and electrophoretic pattern of the components of the histones.

From the findings of this study it was postulated that abnormalities in the biosynthesis of arginine-rich histones might be in-

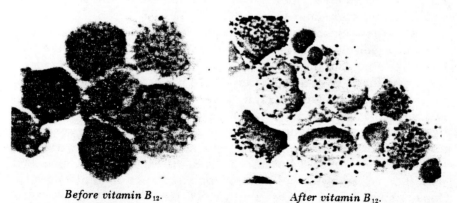

Before vitamin B_{12}.   *After vitamin B_{12}.*

Figure 114. Autoradiographic study of megaloblasts before (left) and after (right) treatment with vitamin B_{12}. Substantial uptake of tritiated arginine into the nucleus can be seen after exposure of the megaloblasts to vitamin B_{12} (right), indicating that an increase in the biosynthesis of arginine-rich histone has occurred. (From Blood 41:549, 1973. Reproduced with permission of Grune & Stratton, New York.)

CONTROL   AFTER B$_{12}$

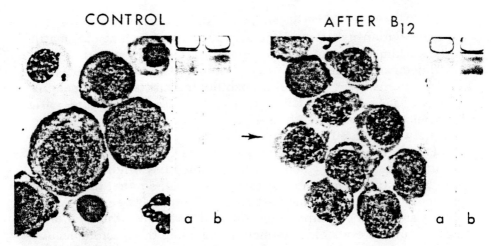

a b   a b

Figure 115. Electrophoretic pattern of pH 1.8 fraction (lysine-rich) and pH 1.0 fraction (arginine-rich) before and after treatment with vitamin B$_{12}$. The pH 1.8 gels are labeled "a" and pH 1.0 gels are labeled "b." Photomicrographs illustrate marrow cells from which the histones in adjacent gels were extracted. The change in marrow cytology from proerythroblasts and aberrant-appearing intermediate and late megaloblasts to intermediate macronormoblasts as a result of exposure of cells to vitamin B$_{12}$ is illustrated. Disappearance of the lower band in the pH 1.8 gel and intensification of the lower band of the pH 1.0 gel are seen in comparing the vitamin B$_{12}$-treated histones to the control, untreated histones. (From *Blood 41*:549, 1973. Reproduced with permission of Grune & Stratton, New York.)

volved in the pathogenesis of megaloblastic erythropoiesis in the following manner. Cytochemically, lysine-rich histones (Plate 2) predominate in the nuclei of pernicious anemia proerythroblasts and megaloblasts.[239] Lysine-rich histones are believed to cause chromatin dispersal.[160] Morphologically, this chromatin dispersal may be reflected in the delicately fenestrated nuclear chromatin pattern of megaloblasts. Arginine-rich histones, lacking substantially in megaloblasts, normally cause aggregation of DNA strands into compact masses of chromatin[160] as found in normoblastic erythroid precursors and in macronormoblastic erythroid precursors after exposure to vitamin B$_{12}$.

The preponderance of lysine-rich histone in untreated megaloblasts and relative lack of arginine-rich histone may cause DNA strands to adhere less tenaciously to one another, producing the thin, elongated strands of nuclear chromatin that are characteristic of the megaloblast. A lack of arginine-rich histone may also be responsible in part for the clockface chromatin pattern observed in pernicious anemia megaloblasts.[238] It is also possible that the decreased numbers of chromatin aggregates in megaloblastic erythroid precursors occur in part as a result of a lack of arginine-rich histone, the basic nucleoprotein that is believed to cement DNA strands into compact aggregates of chromatin.[160]

The fenestrated appearance of the megaloblast nucleus as viewed under the light microscope has been appreciated for many years.[64,110,122,129,133,230-233,241] Based on the studies reviewed above, the apparent widening of the distance between adjacent chromatin strands leading to a fenestrated appearance may be partly due to an actual decrease in the width of DNA strands as a result of defective DNA synthesis.[30-36,260,292] In all probability the filamentous-appearing strands of megaloblastic DNA such as those seen in Figures 107, 108A, and 108B contribute to the light microscope appearance of the delicately fenestrated megaloblast nucleus.

The fenestration may also be partly due to histone abnormalities[239-242] that could lead to defective binding of DNA strands, causing them to appear thin or attenuated rather than coarse and ropelike as in a normoblast. Relationships between DNA and histone are only beginning to be explored on an ultrastructural level and may ultimately yield information regarding the macromolecular configurations and spatial relationships between these two substances.

The pathogenesis of the chromosomal abnormalities in pernicious anemia is uncertain. Aberrant mitotic figures with elongated chromosomes (Fig. 116) are frequent, and chromosomal gaps and constrictions, breaks and fractures, and missing chromosomes have been noted in untreated pernicious anemia by various authors [23,55,152,196,254,290,331] as shown in Figure 117.

Several possible explanations can be offered for these chromosomal abnormalities. Inhibition of DNA synthesis in pernicious anemia[30-36,260,292] may produce chromosomes that are more attenuated and fragile than normal. Beck[30-36] has proposed an unbalanced growth hypothesis to explain these filamentous strands of DNA, and Powsner and Berman[331] have observed that the chromosomes in pernicious anemia are longer than normal, as seen in Figures 116 and

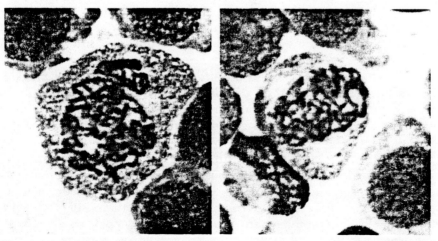

Figure 116. Aberrant mitotic figures in giant erythroid precursor from the bone marrow of a patient with severe pernicious anemia. Elongated and twisted chromosomes are seen.

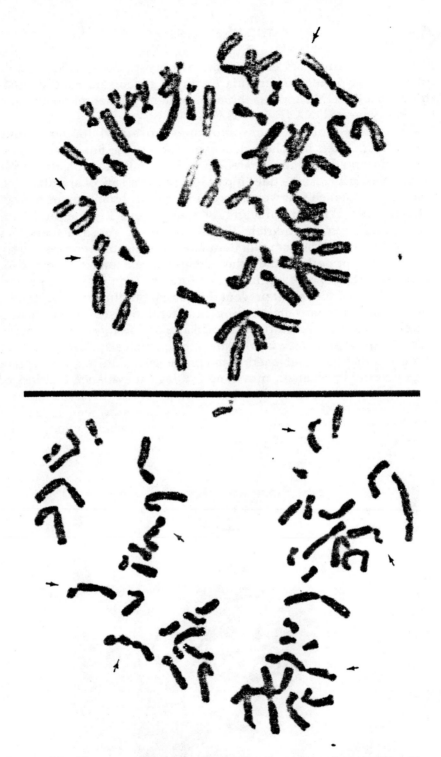

Figure 117. Chromosomal aberrations in erythroid precursors from patients with severe pernicious anemia. Arrows point to areas of focal gaps and constrictions, and chromosomal fragments may also be observed. (From Heath, C. W., Jr., Blood 27:800–815, 1966. Reproduced with permission of C. W. Heath, Jr., M.D., Atlanta, Ga., and Grune & Stratton, New York.)

118. Recent preliminary electron microscopic studies of DNA strands isolated from pernicious anemia erythroid precursors have demonstrated that the DNA appears thinner and more filamentous compared to other types of DNA (Figs. 108A and 108B).

The thin elongated chromosomes observed in pernicious anemia[331] and their morphological expression in the finely attenuated chromatin strands and fenestrated-appearing nuclear chromatin of the megaloblast may also be due in part to a relative lack of arginine-rich histone, a substance that would ordinarily cause chromosomes to form a tight coil.[160] Without sufficient amounts of this histone, and with preponderance of lysine-rich histone known to cause dispersal of chromatin, the chromosomes of pernicious anemia might be less likely to coil tightly or perhaps they may actually have a tendency to uncoil. In either instance, a deficit in arginine-rich histone in untreated pernicious anemia[239,240] might prevent the normal binding of DNA strands and normal chromosomal coiling into tight masses of chromatin, thereby permitting fracture and breakage of chromosomes to occur more readily than otherwise. Figure 118 illustrates such fragments of chromatin that have detached from chromosomes during mitosis in a large erythroid precursor, providing cytological evidence that loss of portions of chromosomes during abnormal mitotic divisions may account for some of the cytogenetic abnormalities as seen in Figure 117.[23,55,152,196,254,290] Some of these "lost" chromosomal fragments may appear as Howell-Jolly bodies.[42,117,224]

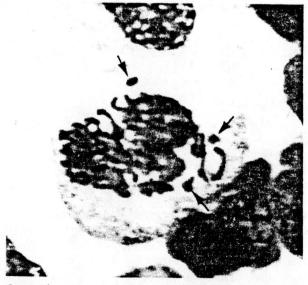

Figure 118.   Large aberrant mitotic figure in erythroid precursor from patient with severe pernicious anemia, showing abnormal karyorrhexis with isolated fragments of chromosomes in the cytoplasm (arrows). These chromosomal fragments are often identifiable as Howell-Jolly bodies.

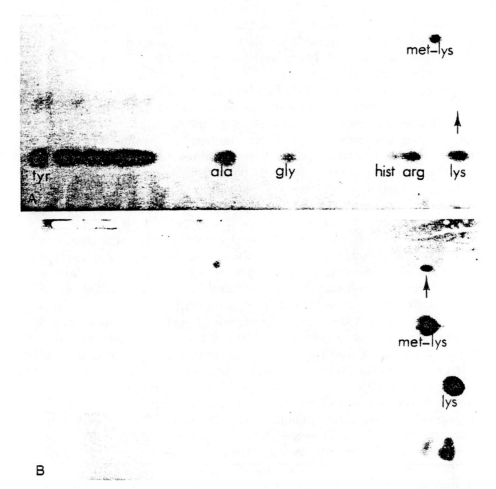

Figure 119. **A.** Electrophoretic pattern of amino acids obtained from pH 1.8 erythroid histone (lysine-rich) prior to vitamin B$_{12}$ therapy. The lysine in the sample (arrow) corresponds in location to the l-lysine in a standard containing a mixture of known amino acids (electrophoretic pattern at the bottom of the figure). (From Blood *44*:125, 1974. Reproduced with permission of Grune & Stratton, New York.) **B.** Electrophoretic pattern of amino acids obtained from pH 1.8 erythroid histone 24 hours after treatment with cyanocobalamin. The majority of the lysine in the sample (arrow) corresponds in mobility to the methyl-l-lysine standard. Scant amounts of l-lysine were also observed in some instances. The electrophoretic pattern at the bottom represents a mixture of l-lysine and methyl-l-lysine as a reference standard. (From Blood *44*:125, 1974. Reproduced with permission of Grune & Stratton, New York.)

A second biochemical study of histones in pernicious anemia may also have bearing on the pathogenesis of megaloblastic erythropoiesis. This study measured acetylation and methylation of histones in pernicious anemia megaloblasts before and after therapy with vitamin B$_{12}$ *in vivo* and *in vitro*.[242] It was observed that both acetylation and methylation of histones increased markedly after exposure of the megaloblasts to vitamin B$_{12}$ and that the labeled acetate radical used in the experiment was incorporated directly into the histone molecule.

In this study it was also found that after exposure to vitamin B_{12} the amino acid lysine in these histones fractions appeared to have been methylated, and methyl-lysine was found on the post-B_{12} histone hydrolysates (Fig. 119).

A possible consequence of abnormalities in histone methylation in pernicious anemia may be the development of gaps and constrictions in chromosomes. Since defects in the methylation of histones are believed to affect mitosis and the integrity of chromosomal structure,[402] the abnormal-appearing mitotic figures in pernicious anemia may be due in part to defects in both DNA synthesis and abnormalities in histone methylation. These abnormalities could contribute to the development of chromosomal gaps and constrictions during abnormal mitotic divisions.

A further consequence of defective methylation of histones in untreated pernicious anemia megaloblasts may be the development of giant, bizarre-appearing erythroid precursors (Fig. 120). The studies of Schleicher,[365] Schwarz,[369] and Berman[41] have suggested that these giant erythroblasts arise in large part as a result of abnormal suppression of cytokinesis. Methylation of histones is believed to be involved in the "events prior to mitosis."[402] Tidwell et al.[402] have proposed that methylation of the epsilon-amino group of lysine in histones may be correlated with the structural and functional changes known to occur in the nucleus prior to mitosis. In pernicious anemia, methylation of histones has been shown to be abnormal, and methylation of lysine in the arginine-rich fraction in particular is defective.[242] As a result of the abnormalities of histone methylation and lysine methylation in pernicious anemia, the "events prior to mitosis" such as maintenance of the mitotic spindle apparatus and uncoiling of chromosomes might be abnormal. These abnormalities could lead to suppression of cytokinesis and the development of gigantic erythroid precursors.[41,365,369]

The consequences of defective acetylation of histones in pernicious anemia are poorly understood. Acetylation of histones apparently causes a change in the fine structure of chromosomes, causing them to bind avidly to acridine orange.[252] As a result of the acetylation of histones, changes in genetic activation are believed to occur, leading to increased RNA synthesis[329] and ultimately to normal mitotic division.

In untreated pernicious anemia megaloblasts, cytoplasmic RNA content is elevated and RNA synthesis is inactive.[260,429] However, after exposure of megaloblasts to vitamin B_{12} and presumably acetylation of histones,[242] there is no evidence that RNA synthesis increases, as might be expected in the process of gene activation. Yet, as observed by Horrigan et al.[216] the macromolecular pattern of RNA as demonstrated with the pyronin stain changes from a block-like configuration to a more diffuse pattern, suggesting that changes in the distribu-

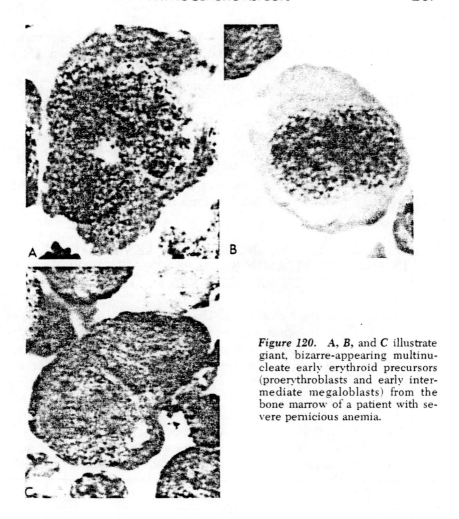

Figure 120. **A, B,** and **C** illustrate giant, bizarre-appearing multinucleate early erythroid precursors (proerythroblasts and early intermediate megaloblasts) from the bone marrow of a patient with severe pernicious anemia.

tion and perhaps the structural configurations of RNA occur as a result of exposure of megaloblasts to vitamin B$_{12}$. In this manner, although the role of histone acetylation in vitamin B$_{12}$ deficiency is ill-defined, it may play a role in RNA metabolism and perhaps ultimately in mitotic division.

From the available evidence, it is likely that a number of factors are involved in the pathogenesis of the morphological lesion of the megaloblast. Defects in DNA synthesis, perhaps the phenomenon of "unbalanced growth" as noted by Beck in the case of vitamin B$_{12}$–deficient *Lactobacillus leichmannii*, and the cytochemical and biochemical abnormalities of histones are probably contributing factors. Possibly a combination of factors including defective DNA synthesis, lack of arginine-rich histone to bind chromosomes into compact coils, preponderance of lysine-rich histone that would tend to cause chromatin dispersal, and abnormalities of histone acetylation and methylation converge to create the finely attenuated chromatin strands and the fenestrated appearance of the pernicious anemia megaloblast nucleus.

In these ways, the original morphological observations of Cabot[64] and of Ehrlich and Lazarus in 1905;[133] who stated that the nucleus of the megaloblast had "a peculiar lack of affinity for the nuclear stains," are beginning to be explored and redefined in the light of newer techniques of nuclear protein and nucleic acid biochemistry and high resolution electron microscopy. With further studies, the mystery of the pathogenesis of the megaloblastic lesion and its continued challenge over the past 96 years may become more fully understood.

PATHOGENETIC IMPLICATIONS OF ABNORMALITIES IN THE TWO VITAMIN B_{12}–DEPENDENT ENZYMES IDENTIFIED THUS FAR IN MAN

Activity of methylmalonyl-CoA mutase, the 5'-deoxyadenosylcobalamin-dependent enzyme responsible for catalyzing the conversion of L-methylmalonyl-CoA to succinyl-CoA, is believed to be reduced in patients with deficiency of vitamin B_{12}.[170,373] One of the anticipated consequences of a deficit of methylmalonyl-CoA mutase or a reduction of its activity might be a metabolic block proximal to the enzyme action. This block would lead to an accumulation of those metabolic intermediates that might normally be converted to succinyl-CoA and ultimately metabolized in the citric acid cycle. Cytochemical evidence for such a metabolic block has recently been suggested in pernicious anemia megaloblasts using the anthraquinone dye alizarine red S.[243] Using this dye to stain megaloblasts on coverslip films of bone marrow fixed in acetate buffered formalin, the cytoplasm of megaloblasts in untreated pernicious anemia stained a unique rose pink color (Plate 2). In treated pernicious anemia, in normal erythroid precursors, and in megaloblasts from patients with severe folate deficiency, the cytoplasmic color was deep yellow. Test tube experiments suggested that one of the major substances responsible for this unusual pink coloration might be methylmalonyl-CoA and that the pink megaloblast might constitute evidence of the metabolic block caused by decreased methylmalonyl-CoA mutase activity.

As a result of the metabolic block and accumulation of methylmalonyl-CoA within the cytoplasm of the megaloblast, alternate pathways for the metabolism of this compound are achieved. Methylmalonicaciduria, described as a characteristic finding in patients with untreated pernicious anemia,[107] is believed to be caused by the deficit in methylmalonyl-CoA mutase activity with consequent accumulation of intracellular methylmalonyl-CoA and its conversion to methylmalonic acid. In some patients with pernicious anemia, the renal excretion of methylmalonic acid as measured by gas chromatographic techniques has been estimated to be as high as 300 micrograms per 24 hours.

Other metabolic intermediates more proximal to the site of activity of the mutase enzyme than methylmalonyl-CoA might also be expected to be abnormally increased in pernicious anemia. This has been noted by Cox et al.[108] who found that there was unusually high excretion of propionic acid in patients with pernicious anemia, ranging from 1.4 to 54.3 milligrams per 24 hours.

Decreased activity of methylmalonyl-CoA mutase may also be involved in the pathogenesis of the neurological manifestations of pernicious anemia. Frenkel[155] has recently demonstrated abnormalities of propionate metabolism in nerve tissue obtained from patients with pernicious anemia. In sural nerve tissue, increased amounts of abnormal fatty acids were found. Since methylmalonyl-CoA mutase is a critical enzyme in the metabolism of propionate, decreased activity of this enzyme in pernicious anemia might be anticipated to cause abnormalities of compounds proximal to methylmalonyl-CoA, including propionate. In this manner, deficits of methylmalonyl-CoA mutase may be involved in the generation of unusual fatty acids in neural tissue and contribute to pathogenesis of some of the nervous system manifestations of pernicious anemia.

N^5-methyltetrahydrofolate-homocysteine methyltransferase enzyme is the second vitamin B_{12}–dependent enzyme identified thus far in man. It contains methylcobalamin as a prosthetic group[279] and is responsible for the conversion of homocysteine to methionine. S-adenosylmethionine is believed to function as a catalyst in the reaction[153,154] and may perhaps be involved in the transient methylation of vitamin B_{12}.[153,154,395] Most evidence to date suggests that N^5-methyltetrahydrofolate is the major methyl donor in the biosynthesis of methionine from homocysteine.[178,179,262,263]

According to the methyltetrahydrofolate trap hypothesis,[49,61,62,201,206,229,313] the enzyme N^5-methyltetrahydrofolate-homocysteine methyltransferase is involved in the synthesis of DNA in the following manner. Decreased activity of the methylcobalamin-dependent methyltransferase in pernicious anemia leads to accumulations of methyltetrahydrofolate and a depletion of other folates necessary for the synthesis of purines and pyrimidines needed for DNA synthesis. DNA synthesis is thereby affected because of the reduction in activity of the methyltransferase enzyme, and the abnormalities in DNA synthesis result in megaloblastic erythropoiesis. It has been postulated that the effects of vitamin B_{12} on DNA are mediated via folate in the manner described,[201,206,292] and to date there has been no evidence demonstrating a direct effect of vitamin B_{12} on DNA synthesis. In fact, the studies of Arnstein[19] have shown that neither vitamin B_{12} nor folate is involved in the methylation of thymine DNA from S-adenosylmethionine.[19,20]

Abnormalities in methylating enzymes and the implications of these abnormalities have only recently been studied.[317] Several studies have indicated that methylation reactions are involved in the metabolism of histones.[317] Methylation of histones has been found to be abnormal in pernicious anemia,[242] and the possible consequences of these abnormalities in methylation have been discussed earlier. They include aberrations in the maintenance of chromatin integrity and in mitotic division, both of which have been considered as dependent in part upon normal methylation of histones.[402] It is uncertain whether methylation of histones is mediated by a vitamin B_{12}– dependent transmethylase, although recently it has been demonstrated that a type of protein methylase not as yet identified as a B_{12}– dependent enzyme preferentially methylates histones rather than a variety of other types of biological substances.[249]

Methylation is also involved in the metabolism of RNA.[329] Although decreases rather than increases in the biosynthesis of RNA have been demonstrated in pernicious anemia megaloblasts after treatment with vitamin B_{12},[429] earlier studies by Horrigan et al.[216] demonstrated that there were changes in the morphological appearance of RNA demonstrated by pyronin staining. The change from block-like RNA aggregates to diffuse staining of RNA may reflect rearrangements of the molecular structure of RNA subsequent to vitamin B_{12} therapy and perhaps as a result of methylating enzymes known to be involved in RNA metabolism. The changes in RNA configurations may also reflect a redistribution of the RNA, unrelated to an effect of a methylating enzyme.

PATHOGENESIS OF THE ANEMIA OF
PERNICIOUS ANEMIA

A number of morphological, erythrokinetic, and cytochemical studies have contributed to our understanding of factors responsible for the anemia of pernicious anemia. From the morphological standpoint, erythrophagocytosis by reticulum cells in lymph nodes was observed by Warthin,[414] and erythrophagocytosis by reticulum cells in the bone marrow of patients with pernicious anemia has been noted by several authors including Cohnheim,[95] Osler and Gardner,[315] and Peabody and Broun.[320] Erythrophagocytosis is believed to constitute cytological evidence for ineffective erythropoiesis, and in the case of pernicious anemia it probably reflects intramedullary destruction of both mature erythrocytes and erythroid precursors (Fig. 121).

Spontaneous degeneration of erythroid precursors within the bone marrow of untreated pernicious anemia patients may also

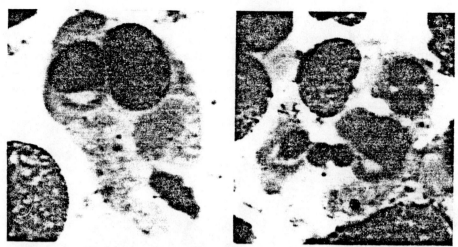

Figure 121. Phagocytosis of mature erythrocytes and degenerating megaloblasts by large histiocytes in the bone marrow of a patient with pernicious anemia. This erythrophagocytosis is cytological evidence of ineffective erythropoiesis. The histiocytes often contain abundant amounts of iron in the form of hemosiderin.

contribute to the development of the anemia. Jedlicka[226] in 1930 was among the first to suggest intramedullary hemolysis of nucleated erythroid cells in this disorder. Lynch and Alfrey[280] demonstrated spontaneous autohemolysis of megaloblastic marrow cells *in vitro* and found that this autohemolysis was considerably greater than that seen in normoblasts.

There are several types of degenerating megaloblasts that may represent morphological evidence for intramedullary destruction of degenerating erythroid precursors in pernicious anemia.[246] One type of degenerating intermediate megaloblast has a vacuous-appearing nucleus with areas seemingly devoid of chromatin strands and cytoplasm that appears homogeneous or vacuolated (Fig. 122, top). A second type of degenerating megaloblast is seen in Figure 122, bottom. The nucleus of this cell appears dense and homogeneous and lacks the usual detail of chromatin strands and aggregates. In addition, the cytoplasm lacks detail and has ragged and disrupted cellular borders. As mentioned earlier, other megaloblasts show evidence of severe defects in hemoglobinization that may further aggravate the anemia.[246] Cytochemically, megaloblasts contain abundant 6-phosphogluconic dehydrogenase, lactic dehydrogenase, and malic dehydrogenase,[385] and it is likely that elevated serum levels of these enzymes derive in part from intramedullary autohemolysis of nucleated erythroid precursors[199,385] as well as from erythrophagocytosis of immature, degenerating erythrocytes and megaloblasts by histiocytic reticulum cells (Fig. 121).

Other metabolic and erythrokinetic studies have also indicated intramedullary destruction of erythroid cells in pernicious anemia. Early studies of bile pigment metabolism in pernicious anemia were performed by Whipple[425,428] in 1922, although at the time Whipple believed that the increased production of stercobilin in pernicious anemia was due to "overproduction" rather than destruction of erythrocytes. London's and West's report[277] demonstrating an "early" stercobilin peak indicated that much of this hyperbilirubinemia was caused by intramedullary destruction of erythrocytes.

According to the studies of Wickramasingehe et al. [431, 432] Cooper

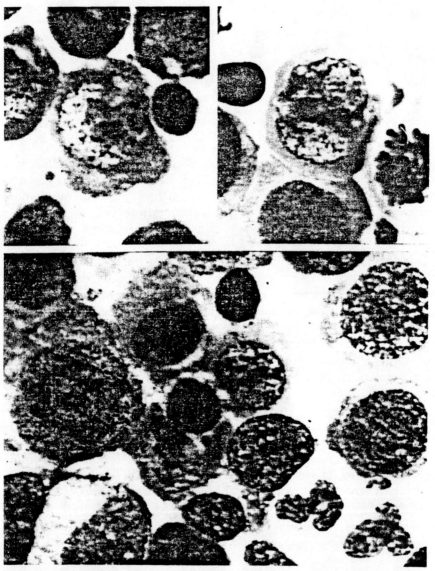

Figure 122. *Top:* degenerating intermediate megaloblasts, severe pernicious anemia, showing vacuous-appearing nuclei and markedly attenuated nuclear chromatin pattern. *Bottom:* several degenerating intermediate megaloblasts with dense-appearing nuclei and ragged-appearing cytoplasm (center).

and Wickramasinghe,[102] and Myhre,[307,308] the cells that may be an important source of the population of erythroid precursors susceptible to intramedullary destruction appear to be the dividing polychromatophilic megaloblasts. These degenerating polychromatophilic intermediate megaloblasts are seen in Figure 122. Wickramasinghe et al.[431-433] found that these abnormal polychromatophilic megaloblasts were increased in number in the G_2 phase, and several cells had DNA contents that were between the 2c and 4c modes and not in DNA synthesis as determined by isotopic labeling. The erythrokinetic studies of Finch et al.[145] and Cronkite et al.[109] demonstrated that the total erythropoietic activity in pernicious anemia was greater than normal, perhaps reflecting the proliferative capacity of the dividing polychromatophilic megaloblast population as studied by Wickramasinghe et al. but that the delivery of viable erythrocytes to the peripheral circulation was less than normal. These factors indicated ineffective erythropoiesis.[109,145]

Abnormalities of iron metabolism may also contribute to the pathogenesis of the anemia of pernicious anemia. As noted in Chapter 2, the serum iron concentration is frequently elevated in untreated pernicious anemia and may be in excess of 200 micrograms percent in some instances. The serum iron binding capacity may be as much as 80% saturated. Cytological evidence of this inability to utilize iron may be found in the bone marrow of patients with untreated pernicious anemia. Figure 123 illustrates megaloblasts stained with the Prussian blue reagent to detect iron. Coarse siderotic granules surrounding the nuclei of the megaloblasts can be seen. These prominent siderotic granules are observed most frequently in the late intermediate megaloblast stage of maturation. Ringed sideroblasts may be found in a variety of other types of anemia, including chronic erythremic myelosis and refractory sideroblastic anemia,[42,244] and perni-

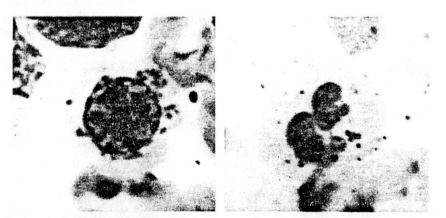

Figure 123. Late intermediate megaloblasts with coarse siderotic granules surrounding the nucleus (ringed sideroblasts) from the bone marrow of a patient with untreated pernicious anemia. Prussian blue stain, neutral red counterstain.

cious anemia may be considered as a type of secondary acquired sideroblastic anemia.

Megaloblasts with coarse ringed siderotic granules reflect the inability of the pernicious anemia erythroid precursors to effectively mobilize and utilize iron. As noted in other types of sideroblastic anemias,[42,244] abnormal iron storage within the erythroid precursor and ensuing abnormalities in iron metabolism may interfere with the normal biosynthesis of hemoglobin, thereby contributing to the pathogenesis of the anemia of pernicious anemia.

In addition to the factors described above, other ill-defined hemolytic factors have been implicated in the pathogenesis of the anemia of pernicious anemia. In 1921, Ashby[21] found that normal donor cells were destroyed rapidly when transfused into untreated pernicious anemia patients. Wearn et al.[417] in 1922 came to similar conclusions in their transfusion studies. The factor(s) responsible for this increased destruction of normal cells after transfusion into pernicious anemia patients are unclear. Hamilton et al.[187] found that if the plasma of untreated pernicious anemia patients was in contact with normal erythrocytes, the survival times of these erythrocytes were substantially decreased when transfused into a normal person, suggesting the possibility of a plasma hemolytic "factor." They also found that the destruction of transfused normal cells was random and irrespective of age when transfused into patients with untreated pernicious anemia.

Other studies indicating abnormal plasma factors in the pathogenesis of the anemia of pernicious anemia have also been reported. These factors were believed to impede the maturation of megaloblasts into more mature erythroid precursors. Astaldi,[22] Lajtha,[258] Callender and Lajtha,[68] and Thompson[399] demonstrated an "inhibitory factor" in the serum of pernicious anemia patients that impeded the normal maturation of megaloblasts into normoblasts in tissue culture. These authors postulated that the inhibition of normal maturation caused by this inhibitory factor could contribute to the development of anemia.

In summary, the anemia of pernicious anemia appears to be due to a combination of interrelating factors. These include erythrophagocytosis by reticulum cells in the bone marrow leading to intramedullary destruction of erythrocytes and erythroid precursors, spontaneous degeneration of megaloblasts within the bone marrow as seen morphologically in the effete-appearing erythroid precursors and perhaps reflected in the elevated serum LDH levels, abnormalities in iron storage and metabolism that may lead to decreased synthesis of hemoglobin, and a particular lability of the dividing polychromatophilic megaloblast population to undergo improper maturation (perhaps in part because of an inhibitory factor) and subsequent destruction leading to ineffective erythropoiesis.

PATHOGENETIC IMPLICATIONS OF THE AUTOIMMUNE ASPECTS OF PERNICIOUS ANEMIA

Although there have been a number of studies demonstrating autoantibodies to intrinsic factor and to parietal cell antigens in virtually all patients with pernicious anemia,[74,205,227] the meaning of these findings in terms of the pathogenesis of pernicious anemia is as yet unclear and controversial. Some authors believe that pernicious anemia may be an autoimmune disorder *per se*,[393] whereas others are willing to concede that immune substances are found in pernicious anemia but that their relationship to the pathogenesis of the disease is uncertain.[205] Still others have not been able to demonstrate a functional role for autoantibodies in pernicious anemia at all.[443]

As noted in Chapter 2, plasma cells in patients with pernicious anemia frequently appear abnormal (Figs. 57, 76, 124, [left]) with multiple large vacuoles and Russell bodies, suggesting that these plasma

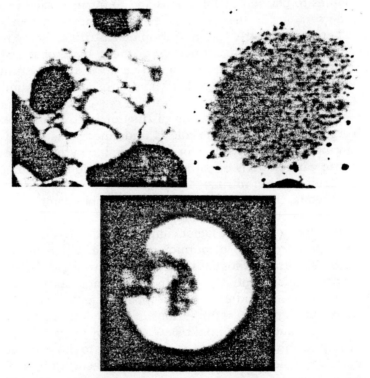

Figure 124. *Above left:* plasma cell with large cytoplasmic vacuoles probably containing immunoglobulins from bone marrow of a patient with untreated pernicious anemia. *Above right:* autoradiograph of plasma cell, untreated pernicious anemia, demonstrating localization of an intrinsic factor-^{60}Co-B$_{12}$ antigen in the cytoplasm. This autoradiographic localization of labeled antigen indicates the presence of an antibody to the intrinsic factor–B$_{12}$ complex in the cytoplasm of the plasma cell. *Below:* plasma cell, untreated pernicious anemia, showing fluorescent antibody localization of a parietal cell antigen conjugated with fluorescein. Intense fluorescence of the plasma cell cytoplasm indicates the presence of parietal cell antibodies.

cells are distended with immunoglobulins and may be actively involved in antibody synthesis. More direct evidence of the ability of
the plasma cells in pernicious anemia to synthesize autoantibodies is
demonstrated in Figure 124. Figure 124, right, illustrates the autoradiographic localization of an intrinsic factor-^{60}Co-B$_{12}$ antigen in the
cytoplasm of plasma cells from a patient with pernicious anemia. The
concentration of isotope in the plasma cell cytoplasm indicates the
presence of antibody to the intrinsic factor–B$_{12}$ complex.

Figure 124, bottom, demonstrates fluorescence of plasma cell
cytoplasm after application of a hog parietal cell antigen conjugated
with fluorescein. The intense fluorescence indicates that antibodies to
parietal cells are contained within the cytoplasm of the plasma cells.
Autoradiographic and immunofluorescent findings such as those described in pernicious anemia plasma cells were not observed either in
plasma cells from normal individuals or from patients with severe
anemia due to folate deficiency.

Antibodies to parietal cell antigens and to intrinsic factor can be
found in the sera and in the gastric juice of patients with pernicious
anemia. Whether the gastric lesion of atrophic gastritis by some means
provokes the production of antibodies to these two substances, or
whether the autoantibodies are produced *de novo* and contribute to
the development of atrophic gastritis and subsequent vitamin B$_{12}$
malabsorption is not known. At this point in our knowledge of these
autoantibodies, one cannot make the distinction with assurance.

Although their pathogenetic role is undefined, it is conceivable
that autoantibodies to intrinsic factor demonstrable in the gastric juice
and in gastric parietal cells of patients with pernicious anemia could
bind to small amounts of intrinsic factor produced by the patient with
pernicious anemia, thereby impeding attachment of vitamin B$_{12}$ to the
intrinsic factor molecule. On the basis of evidence accumulated thus
far, autoantibodies to intrinsic factor cannot as yet be definitely implicated as the primary cause of pernicious anemia. In all probability
they contribute to the pathogenesis of the vitamin B$_{12}$ deficiency by
aggravating the malabsorptive defect in the manner described.

The role of the antibodies to microsomal antigens of parietal cells
in the pathogenesis of the gastric lesions of pernicious anemia is also
uncertain. These antibodies might be capable of aggravating an already existing atrophic gastritis, thus contributing to the pathogenesis
of intrinsic factor deficiency, vitamin B$_{12}$ malabsorption, and consequent development of pernicious anemia.

PATHOGENESIS OF THE NEUROLOGICAL
LESIONS OF PERNICIOUS ANEMIA

Factors leading at first to the diffuse loss of myelin and subsequently axons of the posterior and lateral columns of the spinal

cord[358] and the gray and white matter of the brain[177,440] in pernicious anemia are largely unknown. Numerous studies[6,177,318,440] have shown, however, that in a manner not as yet understood, myelin seems to be the target of the pathological process. Whether it is a primary degeneration of myelin or an abnormality in the maintenance of the integrity of the myelin is not known.

As found by Pant et al.[318] and Greenfield et al.[177] in extensive neuropathological studies, the earliest visible change in the central nervous system in vitamin B_{12} deficiency is a swelling of individual myelinated nerve fibers in small foci. In later stages, the lesions coalesced into larger foci involving many fiber systems. The regions of the cord first and most severely affected were the posterior columns in the cervical and upper thoracic regions. The lesion bore no constant relationship to blood vessels. Fibrillary gliosis was always seen. It appeared as though the largest nerve fibers with the thickest myelin sheaths were the most vulnerable to the deficiency state. In addition to these findings related to the central nervous system, Van der Sheer and Koek[407] also found marked myelin degeneration in the peripheral nerves of patients with pernicious anemia.

Factors that cause swelling of myelinated nerve fibers, loss of myelin, and ultimate disappearance of axons, presumably in part as a result of the loss of myelin, are poorly understood. Several recent studies suggest that decreased activity of methylmalonyl-CoA mutase in pernicious anemia may be related to the pathogenesis of the neurological lesion.[155,411] Methylmalonyl-CoA mutase functions in the propionate pathway of metabolism.[170,373] In pernicious anemia, presumably as a result of the dysfunction of this mutase enzyme, large amounts of methylmalonic acid[107] are found in the urine. Not surprisingly, substantial amounts of propionic acid are also found in the urine, as noted originally by Cox et al.[108] Substantial amounts of acetate are also found in the urine in vitamin B_{12} deficiency,[108] but their relationship to the neuropathological lesions is not understood. The effects of the accumulation of metabolites proximal to the methylmalonyl-CoA mutase have been studied by a number of authors,[170,373] and individuals with a congenital deficiency of this enzyme leading to methylmalonicaciduria have been studied.[373]

Vivacqua et al.[411] were the first to suggest that abnormalities in the propionate pathway might contribute to the pathogenesis of the neurological lesion of pernicious anemia. They found that methylmalonic acid excretion was increased in pernicious anemia, as did Cox et al.,[107] and also noted that the excretion was highest in patients with neurological complications. Injection of ^{14}C-labeled propionate led to excretion of radioactive methylmalonic acid. Autoradiography of a nerve biopsy from a patient receiving radiopropionate was positive for radioactivity. The authors speculated but could not prove conclusively that this radioactivity was due to labeled methylmalonic acid.

They also found that in a patient with pernicious anemia who did not have neurological symptoms, radioactivity was not observed in the nerve biopsy. They postulated that an accumulation of propionate or methylmalonate could be toxic to neural tissue and ultimately lead to a neuropathy.

Recent studies by Frenkel[155] strongly suggest that the dysfunction of methylmalonyl-CoA mutase and consequent accumulation of propionic acid may contribute to the development of the neurological lesion of pernicious anemia as suggested by Vivacqua et al.[411] Frenkel evaluated fatty acid synthesis from radiopropionate in sural nerve biopsy slices from normal persons and nine patients with pernicious anemia. The nerves were incubated in ^{14}C propionate, lipids extracted, and fatty acid methyl esters identified by gas-liquid chromatography.

Frenkel found that in normal nerves the radiolabel was found in the short chain (C_{12} and C_{14}) fatty acids. In pernicious anemia, there were two fatty acid peaks not found in the normals. These were a C_{15} and a C_{17} fatty acid. These two peaks contained the majority of the radioactivity recovered in the fatty acid fractions after incubation with ^{14}C propionate. These were not unsaturated fatty acids. Frenkel also found that the nerves in pernicious anemia had a decrease in the mean content of normal fatty acids and a decrease in the mean synthesis of normal fatty acids compared to normal nerves.

On the basis of Frenkel's studies, one can postulate that a decrease in the activity of methylmalonyl-CoA mutase could lead to the accumulation of propionic acid, as shown by Cox et al.[108] This accumulation of propionate might contribute to the formation of unusual types of fatty acids and decreased synthesis of normal neural fatty acids. As a result of these abnormal types of fatty acids as well as decreased normal fatty acids, myelin integrity might be compromised and subsequently lead to loss of axons, histopathological lesions, neuropathy, and the sensory and motor deficits characteristic of subacute combined degeneration of the spinal cord.

EPILOGUE

The final chapters in the story of pernicious anemia are yet to be written, since many of the original observations made years ago by Ehrlich,[129,133] Hayem,[194,195] Cohnheim,[95] Osler,[315,316] and Cabot[64-66] are still unexplained:

Why does the megaloblast show nucleocytoplasmic asynchrony?

What are the biochemical and biophysical abnormalities that cause the chromatin of the megaloblast to appear fenestrated?

Why should a deficiency of an essential vitamin cause a cell to increase in size, sometimes to dramatic proportions?

Are there other as yet unidentified enzyme systems in man that are vitamin B_{12}–dependent?

What is the relationship of vitamin B_{12} to the larger problem of neoplasia and carcinogenesis, particularly in the DiGuglielmo syndrome in which megaloblastoid erythroid precursors superficially resemble megaloblasts as found in pernicious anemia?

Do these megaloblastoid erythroid precursors in a preleukemic disorder of erythropoiesis have an abnormality or abnormalities of a vitamin B_{12}–dependent enzyme system or systems?

Until the answers to these and other questions are found, the megaloblast whose nucleus has a "much less marked affinity for the nuclear stains"[133] and the red crystalline needles of vitamin B_{12} [345,376] whose properties have only begun to be understood, beckon investigators onward in what seems to be the continuing challenge of pernicious anemia.

REFERENCES

1. Abeles, R. H. and Zagalak, B. The nature of the hydrogen transfer in the dimethyl-benzimidazolylcobamide coenzyme-catalyzed conversion of 1,2 propanediol to propionaldehyde. J. Biol. Chem. 241:1245, 1966.
2. Abels, J. and Schilling, R. F. Protection of intrinsic factor by vitamin B_{12}. J. Lab. Clin. Med. 64:375, 1964.
3. Ackerman, A. and Bellios, N. C. A study of the morphology of the living cells of blood and bone marrow in supravital films with the phase contrast microscope. Blood 10:1183, 1955.
4. Adami, J. G. Latent infection and subinfection and the etiology of hemochromatosis and pernicious anemia. Med. News 76:8, 1900.
5. Adams, J. F., Glen, A. I. M., Kennedy, E. H., MacKenzie, I. L., Morrow, J. M., Anderson, J. R., Gray, K. G., and Middleton, D. G. The histological and secretory changes in the stomach in patients with autoimmunity to gastric parietal cells. Lancet 1:401, 1964.
6. Adams, J. M. and McQuarrie, I. Severe functional anemia in a child resembling pernicious anemia of adults. J. Pediat. 12:176, 1938.
7. Adams, R. D. and Kubik, C. S. Subacute degeneration of the brain in pernicious anemia. New Eng. J. Med. 231:1, 1944.
8. Addison, T. Anaemia—disease of the supra-renal capsules. London Med. Gaz. 43:517, 1849.
9. Addison, T. On the Constitutional and Local Effects of Disease of the Supra-renal Capsules. Samuel Highley, London, 1855.
10. Alsted, G. Pernicious anaemia after nitric acid corrosion of the stomach. Lancet 1:76, 1937.
11. Andreasen, J. P. Anaemia perniciosa hos et 14 aars barn. Ugeskr. Laeg. 103:783, 1941.
12. Ardeman, S., Chanarin, I., and Doyle, J. C. Studies on secretion of gastric intrinsic factor in man. Brit. Med. J. 2:600, 1964.
13. Ardeman, S., Chanarin, I., and Berry, V. Studies on human gastric intrinsic factor. Observations on its possible absorption and enterohepatic circulation. Brit. J. Haemat. 11:11, 1965.
14. Ardeman, S. and Chanarin, I. Intrinsic factor antibodies and intrinsic factor mediated vitamin B_{12} absorption in pernicious anemia. Gut 6:436, 1965.
15. Ardeman, S. and Chanarin, I. Steroids and Addisonian pernicious anemia. New Eng. J. Med. 273:1352, 1965.
16. Ardeman, S. and Chanarin, I. Gastric intrinsic factor after partial gastrectomy. Gut 7:217, 1966.
17. Arinkin, M. I. Die intravitale Untersuchungsmethodik des Knochenmarks. Folia Haemat. 38:233, 1929.
18. Arneth, J. Diagnose und Therapie der Anämien. Stuber, Würzburg, 1907, p. 61.
19. Arnstein, H. R. V. and White, A. M. The function of vitamin B_{12} in the metabolism of propionate by the protozoan Ochromonas malhamensis. Biochem. J. 83:264, 1962.

220

20. Arnstein, H. R. V. The metabolic functions of folic acid and vitamin B_{12}. Ser. Haemat. 3:38, 1965.

21. Ashby, W. Study of transfused blood. II. Blood destruction in pernicious anemia. J. Exp. Med. 34:147, 1921.

22. Astaldi. G. Differentiation, proliferation and maturation of haematopoietic cells studied in tissue culture. In Ciba Foundation Symposium on Haemopoiesis: Cell Production and its Regulation, Wolstenholme, G. E. W. and O'Connor, M., eds. Little, Brown & Co., Boston, 1960, p. 99.

23. Astaldi, G., Strosselli, E., and Airò, R. Ricerche citogenetiche nelle emopatie. Osservazioni sui cromosomi dell' anemia perniciosa non trattata 1) alterazioni numeriche. Boll. Soc. Ital. Biol. Sper. 38:111, 1962.

24. Astaldi, G., Strosselli, E., and Airò, R. Ricerche citogenetiche nelle emopatie. Osservazioni sui cromosomi dell' anemia perniciosa non trattata 2) alterazioni morfologiche. Boll. Soc. Ital. Biol. Sper. 38:114, 1962.

25. Astaldi, G., Strosselli, E., Airò, R., and Pollini, G. Recherches cytogénétiques dans l'anémie pernicieuse après traitment. Schweiz. Med. Wschr. 92:1332, 1962.

26. Barclay, A. W. Death from anaemia. Med. Times Gaz. 23:480, 1851.

27. Barker, H. A., Weissbach, H., and Smyth, R. D. A coenzyme containing pseudovitamin B_{12}. Proc. Nat. Acad. Sci. USA 44:1093, 1958.

28. Baur, S., Fisher, J. M., Strickland, R. G., and Taylor, K. B. Autoantibody-containing cells in the gastric mucosa in pernicious anemia. Lancet 2:887, 1968.

29. Beard, M. F., Pitney, W. P., and Sanneman, E. H. Serum concentrations of vitamin B_{12} in patients suffering from leukemia. Blood 9:789, 1954.

30. Beck, W. S. Metabolic functions of vitamin B_{12}: The possible relationship of megaloblast formation to unbalanced growth in bacteria requiring vitamin B_{12}. J. Clin. Invest. 40:1024, 1961.

31. Beck, W. S., Goulian, M., and Hook, S. The metabolic functions of vitamin B_{12}. II. Participation of vitamin B_{12} in the biosynthesis of deoxyribonucleic acid and its acid soluble precursors. Biochim. Biophys. Acta 55:470, 1962.

32. Beck, W. S., Hook, S., and Barnett, B. H. The metabolic functions of vitamin B_{12}. I. Distinctive modes of unbalanced growth behavior in Lactobacillus leichmannii. Biochim. Biophys. Acta 55:455, 1962.

33. Beck, W. S. The metabolic basis of megaloblastic erythropoiesis. Medicine 43:715, 1964.

34. Beck, W. S. Deoxyribonucleotide synthesis and the role of vitamin B_{12} in erythropoiesis. Vitam. Horm. 26:413, 1968.

35. Beck, W. S. General considerations of megaloblastic anemias. In Hematology, Williams, W. J. et al., eds. McGraw-Hill, New York, 1972, p. 249.

36. Beck, W. S. Vitamin B_{12} deficiency. In Hematology, Williams, W. J. et al., eds. McGraw-Hill. New York, 1972, p. 256.

37. Becker, G. Liver treatment in diseases with a bloodpicture of pernicious anemia. Acta Med. Scand. Suppl. 34:70, 1930.

38. Benjamin, B. Infantile form of pernicious (Addisonian) anemia. Amer. J. Dis. Child. 75:143,1948.

39. Bennett, M. A., Joralemon, J., and Halpern, P. E. The effect of vitamin B_{12} on rat growth and fat infiltration of the liver. J. Biol. Chem. 193:285, 1957.

40. Berlin, R., Berlin, H., Brante, G., and Sjöberg, S. G. Failures in long-term oral treatment of pernicious anemia with B_{12}–intrinsic factor preparations. Acta Med. Scand. 161:143, 1958.

41. Berman, L. The clinical significance of cellular gigantism in human erythropoiesis. J. Lab. Clin. Med. 32:793, 1947.

42. Bessis, M. Living Blood Cells and Their Ultrastructure. Springer Verlag, New York, 1973.

43. Bethell, F. H., Swendseid, M. E., Bird, O. D., Brown, R. A., Meyers, M. C., and Andrews, G. A. Further studies on the utilization of pteroyl hexa-glutamyl glutamic acid (vitamin B_c conjugate) in pernicious anemia. Proc. Cent. Soc. Clin. Res. 19:28 Nov., 1946.

44. Biermer, A. Tageblatt der 42. Versammlung Deutscher Naturforscher und Aerzte in Dresden vom 18 bis 24 September 1868. Druck und Verlag von B. G. Teubner, Dresden, 1868, p. 173.

45. Biermer, A. Hält Zunächst einen Vortrag über eine von ihm öfters beobachtete eigenthümliche Form von progressiver perniziöser Anämie. Corresp. Schweiz. Aerzte 2:15, 1872.

46. Billings, F. The changes in the spinal cord and medulla in pernicious anemia. Boston Med. Surg. J. *147*:225, 1902.

47. Bishop R. C., Toporek, M., Nelson, N. A., and Bethell, F. H. The relationship of binding power to intrinsic factor activity. J. Lab. Clin. Med. *46*:796, 1955.

48. Blackburn, E. K., Cohen, H., and Wilson, G. M. Oral treatment of pernicious anaemia with a combined vitamin B_{12} and intrinsic factor preparation. Brit. Med. J. *2*:461, 1955.

49. Blakley, R. L. *The Biochemistry of Folic Acid and Related Pteridines*. Frontiers of Biology, vol. 13. North Holland, Amsterdam, 1969, ch. 13, p. 439.

50. Bloomfield, A. L. and Keefer, C. S. Clinical studies of gastric function. J. Amer. Med. Ass. *88*:707, 1927.

51. Bock, H. E., Hartje, J., Müller, D., and Wilmanns, W. Thyminnucleotid-Synthese und Proliferation von Knochenmarkzellen bei megaloblastären Anämien unter der Einwirkung von Vitamin B_{12}. Klin. Wschr. *45*:176, 1967.

52. Bonnett, R., Cannon, J. R., Johnson, A. W., Sutherland, I., Todd, A. R., and Smith, E. L. The structure of vitamin B_{12} and its hexacarboxylic acid degradation product. Nature *176*:328, 1955.

53. Booth, C. C. and Mollin, D. L. Plasma, tissue, and urinary radioactivity after oral administration of ^{56}Co-labelled vitamin B_{12}. Brit. J. Haemat. *2*:223, 1956.

54. Booth, C. C. and Mollin, D. L. The site of absorption of vitamin B_{12} in man. Lancet *1*:18, 1959.

55. Bottura, C. and Coutinho, V. The chromosome anomalies of the megaloblastic anaemias. Blut *16*:193, 1968.

56. Bowman, H. M. On the association of disease of the spinal cord with pernicious anaemia. Brain *17*:198, 1894.

57. Bramwell, B. The clinical features of myxoedema. Edinburgh Med. J. *38*:985, 1893.

58. Bramwell, B. Clinical Studies. II. On the association of pernicious anaemia with subacute combined degeneration of the spinal cord. Edinburgh Med. J. *14* n.s.:260, 1915.

59. Brody, E. A., Estren, S., and Herbert, V. Coexistent pernicious anemia and malabsorption in four patients including one whose malabsorption disappeared with vitamin B_{12} therapy. Ann. Int. Med. *64*:1246, 1966.

60. Brown, M. A., Langdon, F. W., and Wolfstein, D. I. Combined sclerosis of Lichtheim-Putnam-Dana type accompanying pernicious anemia. J. Amer. Med. Ass. *36*:552, 1901.

61. Buchanan, J. M., Elford, H. L., Loughlin, R. E., McDougall, B. M., and Rosenthal, S. The role of vitamin B_{12} in methyl transfer to homocysteine. Ann. N.Y. Acad. Sci. *112*:756, 1964.

62. Buchanan, J. M. The function of vitamin B_{12} and folic acid coenzymes in mammalian cells. Medicine *43*:697, 1964.

63. Bunge, M. B. and Schilling, R. F. Intrinsic factor studies. VI. Competition for vit. B_{12} binding sites offered by analogues of the vitamin. Proc. Soc. Exp. Biol. Med. *96*:587, 1957.

64. Cabot, R. C. *A Guide to the Clinical Examination of the Blood for Diagnostic Purposes*. 3rd revised edition. W. Wood & Co., New York, 1898.

65. Cabot, R. C. Pernicious anaemia: a study of one hundred and ten cases. Amer. J. Med. Sci. *120*:139, 1900.

66. Cabot, R. C. Ring bodies (nuclear remnants?) in anemic blood. J. Med. Res. *9*:15, 1903.

67. Cahn, A. and von Mering, J. Die Säuren des gesunden und kranken Magens. Deutsch. Arch. Klin. Med. *39*:233, 1886.

68. Callender, S. T. and Lajtha, L. G. On the nature of Castle's hemopoietic factor. Blood *6*:1234, 1951.

69. Callender, S. T., Retief, F. P., and Witts, L. J. The augmented histamine test with special reference to achlorhydria. Gut *1*:326, 1960.

70. Camp, C. D. Pernicious anemia causing spinal cord changes and a mental state resembling paresis. Med. Rec. *81*:156, 1912.

71. Cannata, J. J. B., Focesi, A., Mazumder, R., Warner, R. C., and Ochoa, S. Metabolism of propionic acid in animal tissues. XII. Properties of mammalian methylmalonyl coenzyme A mutase. J. Biol. Chem. *240*:3249, 1965.

72. Capps, J. A. A study of volume index. Observations upon the volume of erythrocytes in various disease conditions. J. Med. Res. *10*:367, 1903.
73. Cardinale, G. J. and Abeles, R. H. Mechanistic similarities in the reactions catalyzed by dioldehydrase and methylmalonyl-CoA mutase. Biochim. Biophys. Acta *132*:517, 1967.
74. Carmel, R. and Herbert, V. Presence of "precipitating" or "blocking" antibody to intrinsic factor in gastric juice or serum of nearly all pernicious anemia patients. Clin. Res. *14*:482, 1966 (abstract).
75. Carmel, R. and Herbert, V. Correctable intestinal defect of vitamin B_{12} absorption in pernicious anemia. Ann. Int. Med. *67*:1201, 1967.
76. Carmel, R. and Herbert V. Intrinsic-factor antibody in the saliva of a patient with pernicious anaemia. Lancet *1*:80, 1967.
77. Carmel, R., Rosenberg, A. H., Lau, K.-S., Streiff, R. R., and Herbert, V. Vitamin B_{12} uptake by human small bowel homogenate and its enhancement by intrinsic factor. Gastroenterology *56*:548, 1969.
78. Castle, W. B. and Locke, E. A. Observations on the etiological relationship of achylia gastrica to pernicious anemia. J. Clin. Invest. *6*:2, 1928 (abstract).
79. Castle, W. B. Observations on the etiologic relationship of achylia gastrica to pernicious anemia. I. The effect of the administration to patients with pernicious anemia of the contents of the normal human stomach recovered after the ingestion of beef muscle. Amer. J. Med. Sci. *178*:748, 1929.
80. Castle, W. B. and Townsend, W. C. Observations on the etiologic relationship of achylia gastrica to pernicious anemia. II. The effect of the administration to patients with pernicious anemia of beef muscle after incubation with normal human gastric juice. Amer. J. Med. Sci. *178*:764, 1929.
81. Castle, W. B., Townsend, W. C., and Heath, C. W. Observations on the etiologic relationship of achylia gastrica to pernicious anemia. III. The nature of the reaction between normal human gastric juice and beef muscle leading to clinical improvement and increased blood formation similar to the effect of liver feeding. Amer. J. Med. Sci. *180*:305, 1930.
82. Castle, W. B., Heath, C. W., and Strauss, M. Observations on the etiologic relationship of achylia gastrica to pernicious anemia. IV. A biologic assay of the gastric secretion of patients with pernicious anemia having free hydrochloric acid and that of patients without anemia or with hypochromic anemia having no free hydrochloric acid, and of the role of intestinal impermeability to hematopoietic substances in pernicious anemia. Amer. J. Med. Sci. *182*:741, 1931.
83. Castle, W. B. and Ham, T. H. Observations on the etiologic relationship of achylia gastrica to pernicious anemia. V. Further evidence for the essential participation of extrinsic factor in hematopoietic responses to mixtures of beef muscle and gastric juice and to hog stomach mucosa. J. Amer. Med. Assoc. *107*:1456, 1936.
84. Castle, W. B. Development of knowledge concerning the gastric intrinsic factor and its relation to pernicious anemia. New Eng. J. Med. *249*:603, 1953.
85. Castle, W. B. Factors involved in the absorption of vitamin B_{12}. Gastroenterology *37*:377, 1959.
86. Castle, W. B. Current concepts of pernicious anemia. Amer. J. Med. *48*:541, 1970.
87. Chaiet, L., Rosenblum, C., and Woodbury, D. T. Biosynthesis of radioactive vitamin B_{12} containing cobalt[60]. Science *111*:601, 1950.
88. Chanarin, I. *The Megaloblastic Anaemias.* Blackwell Scientific, Oxford, England, 1969.
89. Chanarin, I. Cobalamin and folate interrelationships. In *The Cobalamins*, Arnstein, H. R. V. and Wrighton, R. J., eds. Churchill Livingstone, Edinburgh, 1971, p. 94.
90. Channing, W. Notes on anhaemia, principally in its connections with the puerperal state, and with functional disease of the uterus; with cases. New Eng. Quart. J. Med. Surg. *1*:157, 1842.
91. Charcot, M. Myxoedème cachexie pachydermique ou ètat crétinoïde. Gaz. des Hop. *54*:73, 1881.
92. Clarke, J. M. On the spinal cord degenerations in anaemia. Brain *27*:441, 1904.
93. Cohen, H. Optic atrophy as the presenting sign in pernicious anaemia. Lancet *2*:1202, 1936.

94. Cohn, E. J., Minot, G. R., Alles, G. A., and Salter, W. T. The nature of the material in liver effective in pernicious anemia. J. Biol. Chem. 77:325, 1928.

95. Cohnheim, J. Erkrankung des Knochenmarkes bei perniciöser Anämie. Arch. Path. Anat. Physiol. Klin. Med. 68:291, 1876.

96. Combe, J. S. History of a case of anaemia. Trans. Med. Chir. Soc. Edinburgh 1:194, 1824. (Presented May 1, 1822.)

97. Cooke, W. E. The macropolycyte. Brit. Med. J. 1:12, 1927.

98. Cooper, B. A. and Castle, W. B. Sequential mechanisms in the enhanced absorption of vitamin B_{12} by intrinsic factor in the rat. J. Clin. Invest. 39:199, 1960.

99. Cooper, B. A. and Paranchych, W. Selective uptake of specifically bound cobalt-58 vitamin B_{12} by human and mouse tumor cells. Nature 191:393, 1961.

100. Cooper, B. A. and White, J. J. Absence of intrinsic factor from human portal plasma during $^{57}CoB_{12}$ absorption in man. Brit. J. Haemat. 14:73, 1968.

101. Cooper, B. A. Complex of intrinsic factor and B_{12} in human ileum during vitamin B_{12} absorption. Amer. J. Physiol. 214:832, 1968.

102. Cooper, E. H. and Wickramasinghe, S. N. Quantitative cytochemistry in the study of erythropoiesis. Ser. Haemat. n.s. II (No. 4):65, 1969.

103. Corcino, J. J., Waxman, S., and Herbert, V. Absorption and malabsorption of vitamin B_{12}. Amer. J. Med. 48:562, 1970.

104. Cornell, B. S. Pernicious Anemia. Duke University Press, Durham, N.C., 1927.

105. Coupland, S. Pernicious Anemia. In A System of Medicine, Allbutt, T. C., ed. Macmillan Co., London, Vol. 5, 1898, p. 519.

106. Courville, C. B. and Nielsen, J. M. Optic atrophy associated with subacute combined degeneration of the spinal cord. Bull. Los Angeles Neurol. Soc. 3:83, 1938.

107. Cox, E. V. and White, A. M. Methylmalonic acid excretion: an index of vitamin B_{12} deficiency. Lancet 2:853. 1962.

108. Cox, E. V., Robertson-Smith, D., Small, M., and White, A. M. The excretion of propionate and acetate in vitamin B_{12} deficiency. Clin. Sci. 35:123, 1968.

109. Cronkite, E. P., Fliedner, T. M., Stryckmans, P., Chanana, A. D., Cuttner, J., and Ramos, J. Flow patterns and rates of human erythropoiesis and granulocytopoiesis. Ser. Haemat. 5:51, 1965.

110. Dacie, J. V. and White, J. C. Erythropoiesis with particular reference to its study by biopsy of human bone marrow. J. Clin. Path. 2:1, 1949.

111. Dameshek, W. and Valentine, E. H. The sternal marrow in pernicious anemia. Arch. Path. 23:159, 1937.

112. Davis, B. D. and Mingioli, E. S. Mutants of Escherichia coli requiring methionine or vitamin B_{12}. J. Bact. 60:17, 1950.

113. Davison, C. Subacute combined degeneration of the cord. Arch. Neurol. and Psychiat. 26:1195,1931.

114. Dedichen, J. Anémie à type pernicieux chez un enfant de 9 mois. Acta Med. Scand. 111:90, 1942.

115. Deller, D. J. and Witts, L. J. Changes in the blood after partial gastrectomy with special reference to vitamin B_{12}. Quart. J. Med. n.s. 31:71, 1962.

116. Dickerman, H., Redfield, B. G., Bieri, J. G., and Weissbach, H. The role of vitamin B_{12} in methionine synthesis in avian liver. J. Biol. Chem. 239:2545, 1964.

117. Discombe, G. L'origine des corps de Howell-Jolly et des anneaux de Cabot. Sang 19:262, 1948.

118. Doig, A., Girdwood, R. H., Duthie, J. J. R., and Knox, J. D. E. Response of megaloblastic anaemia to prednisolone. Lancet 2:966, 1957.

119. Donaldson, R. M., Mackenzie, I. L., and Trier, J. S. Intrinsic factor-mediated attachment of vitamin B_{12} to brush borders and microvillous membranes of hamster intestine. J. Clin. Invest. 46:1215, 1967.

120. Donohue, D. M. and Azzam, S. A. Incorporation of H^3 thymidine and H^3 deoxyuridine into the DNA of bone marrow from patients with pernicious anemia. Clin. Res. 10:108, 1962 (abstract).

121. Doscherholmen, A. and Hagen, P. S. Delay of absorption of radiolabelled cyanocobalamin in the intestinal wall in the presence of intrinsic factor. J. Lab. Clin. Med. 54:434, 1959.

122. Downey, H. The megaloblast-normoblast problem: a cytologic study. J. Lab. Clin. Med. 39:837, 1952.

123. Draper, G. *Human Constitution. A Consideration of its Relationship to Disease.* W. B. Saunders, Philadelphia, 1924.
124. du Vigneaud, V., Dyer, H. M., and Kies, M. W. A relationship between the nature of the vitamin B complex supplement and the ability of homocystine to replace methionine in the diet. J. Biol. Chem. *130*:325, 1939.
125. Eckman, P. F. and Rowe, O. W. Pernicious anemia in a boy aged eleven. Minnesota Med. *12*:788, 1929.
126. Eggerer, H., Stadtmann, E. R., Overath, P., and Lynen, F. Zum Mechanismus der durch Cobalamin-Coenzym katalysierten Umlagerung von Methylmalonyl-CoA in Succinyl-CoA. Biochem. Z. *333*:1, 1960.
127. Eggerer, H., Overath, P., Lynen, F., and Stadtman, E. R. On the mechanism of the cobamide coenzyme dependent isomerization of methylmalonyl CoA to succinyl CoA. J. Amer. Chem. Soc. *82*:2643, 1960.
128. Ehrlich, P. Über die specifischen Granulationen des Blutes. Arch. Anat. Physiol. Phys. Abth. p. 571, 1879.
129. Ehrlich, P. Über Regeneration und Degeneration rother Blutscheiben bei Anämien. Berlin Klin. Wschr. 12 July #28, vol. 117, 1880, p. 405.
130. Ehrlich, P. Beobachtungen über einen Fall von perniziöser, progressiver Anämie mit Sarcombildung. Beiträge zur Lehre von der acuten Herzinsufficienz. Charite-Ann. *5*:198, 1880.
131. Ehrlich, P. Über einige Beobachtungen am anämischen Blut. (Presented on December 9, 1880.) Berlin Klin. Wschr. *18*:43, 1881.
132. Ehrlich, P. Zur Physiologie und Pathologie der Blutscheiben. Charite-Ann. *10*:136, 1885.
133. Ehrlich, P. and Lazarus, A. Anemia. Histology of the blood. Normal and pathologic. In *Diseases of the Blood*, Stengel, A., ed. W. B. Saunders, Philadelphia, 1905, p.17.
134. Eichhorst, H. Ueber die Diagnose der progressiven perniziösen Anämie. Cent. Med. Wissen. *14*:465, 1876.
135. Eichhorst, H. *Die progressive perniziöse Anämie.* von Veit, Leipzig, 1878.
136. Eisenlohr, C. Blut und Knochenmark bei progressiver perniziöser Anämie und bei Magencarcinom. Deutsch. Arch. Klin. Med. *20*:495, 1877.
137. Ellenbogen, L. and Williams, W. L. Quantitative assay of intrinsic factor activity by urinary excretion of radioactive vitamin B_{12}. Blood *13*:582, 1958.
138. Emery, E. S. The blood in myxedema. Amer. J. Med. Sci. *165*:577, 1923.
139. Epstein, R. D. Cells of the megakaryocyte series in pernicious anemia in particular, the effect of specific therapy. Amer. J. Path. *25*:239, 1949.
140. Falabella, F., Hamilton, H. E., Hogenkamp, H. P. C., and Sheets, R. F. Differences in response of megaloblastic marrow cultures to cyano-, methyl-, and 5'-deoxyadenosylcobalamin. J. Lab. Clin. Med. *74*:870, 1969.
141. Fantes, K. H., Page, J. E., Parker, L. F. J., and Smith, E. L. Crystalline antipernicious anaemia factor from liver. Proc. Roy. Soc. Lond. Series B. *136*:592, 1950.
142. Farrant, P. C. Nuclear changes in oral epithelium in pernicious anaemia. Lancet *1*:830, 1958.
143. Feinmann, E. L., Sharp, J., and Wilkinson, J. F. Observations on the behaviour of erythroblasts cultured in normal and "pernicious anaemia" sera. Brit. Med. J. *2*:14, 1952.
144. Fenwick, S. On atrophy of the stomach. Lancet *2*:78, 1870.
145. Finch, C. A., Coleman, D. H., Motulsky, A. G., Donohue, D. M., and Reiff, R. H. Erythrokinetics in pernicious anemia. Blood *11*:807, 1956.
146. Fisher, J. M. and Taylor, K. B. A comparison of autoimmune phenomena in pernicious anemia and chronic atrophic gastritis. New Eng. J. Med. *272*:499, 1965.
147. Fisher, J. M., Rees, C., and Taylor, K. B. Intrinsic factor antibodies in gastric juice of pernicious anaemia patients. Lancet *2*:88, 1966.
148. Fisher, J. M. and Taylor, K. B. The intracellular localization of Castle's intrinsic factor by an immunofluorescent technique using autoantibodies. Immunology *16*:779, 1969.
149. Flint, A. A clinical lecture on anaemia. Amer. Med. Times *1*:181, 1860.
150. Fontana, L. Osservazioni sul midollo osseo esaminato in vivo in casi di anemia perniciosa. Arch. Sci. Med. *52*:497, 1928.

151. Foroozan, P. and Trier, J. S. Mucosa of the small intestine in pernicious anemia. New Eng. J. Med. 277:553, 1967.
152. Forteza Bover, G. and Báguena Candela, R. Analysis cytogenitico de un caso de anemia perniciosa antes y despues del tratamiento. Rev. Clin. Esp. 88:251, 1963.
153. Foster, M. A., Jones, K. M., and Woods, D. D. The purification and properties of a factor containing vitamin B₁₂ concerned in the synthesis of methionine by Escherichia coli. Biochem. J. 80:519, 1961.
154. Foster, M. A., Dilworth, M. J., and Woods, D. D. Cobalamin and the synthesis of methionine by Escherichia coli. Nature 201:39, 1964.
155. Frenkel, E. P. Abnormal fatty acid metabolism in peripheral nerves of patients with pernicious anemia. J. Clin. Invest. 52:1237, 1973.
156. Frey, P. A., Essenberg, M. K., and Abeles, R. H. Studies on the mechanism of hydrogen transfer in the cobamide coenzyme-dependent dioldehydrase reaction. J. Biol. Chem. 242:5369, 1967.
157. Fudenberg, H. and Estren, S. Non-Addisonian megaloblastic anemia. The intermediate megaloblast in the differential diagnosis of pernicious and related anemias. Amer. J. Med. 25:198, 1958.
158. Funke, O. Ueber das Milzvenenblut. Z. Rat. Med. n.f. 1:172, 1851.
159. Gáspár, S. Untersuchungen über Urspung, Zahl und Form der Blutplättchen und über das Benehmen der Knochenmarksriesenzellen (Megakaryozyten) unter normalen und pathologischen Verhältnissen. Frankfurt Z. Path. 34:460, 1926.
160. Gershey, E. L., Haslett, G. W., Vidali, G., and Allfrey, V. G. Chemical studies of histone methylation. Evidence for the occurrence of 3-methylhistidine in avian erythrocyte histone fractions. J. Biol. Chem. 244:4871, 1969.
161. Girdwood, R. H. The interrelationships of factors that influence the megaloblastic anemias. Blood 7:77, 1952.
162. Glass, G. B. J., Boyd, L. J., Rubinstein, M. A., and Svigals, C. S. Relationship of glandular mucoprotein from human gastric juice to Castle's intrinsic antianemic factor. Science 115:101, 1952.
163. Glass, G. B. J. Scintillation measurements of the uptake of radioactive vitamin B₁₂ by the liver in normal humans and patients with pernicious and other macrocytic anemias. Bull. N. Y. Acad. Med. Series 2. 30:717, 1954.
164. Glass, G. B. J. Gastric intrinsic factor and its function in the metabolism of vitamin B₁₂. Physiol. Rev. 43:529, 1963.
165. Glazer, H. S., Mueller, J. F., Jarrold, T., Sakurai, K., Will, J. J., and Vilter, R. W. The effect of vitamin B₁₂ and folic acid on nucleic acid composition of the bone marrow of patients with megaloblastic anemia. J. Lab. Clin. Med. 43:905, 1954.
166. Goldhamer, S. M., Bethell, F. H., Isaacs, R., and Sturgis, C. C. The occurrence and treatment of neurologic changes in pernicious anemia. J. Amer. Med. Ass. 103:1663, 1934.
167. Goldhamer, S. M. The presence of the intrinsic factor of Castle in the gastric juice of patients with pernicious anemia. Amer. J. Med. Sci. 191:405, 1936.
168. Goldhamer, S. M. Macrocytic anemia in cancer of the stomach, apparently due to lack of intrinsic factor. Amer. J. Med. Sci. 195:17, 1938.
169. Goldstein, H. I. Biermerin or Addisonin in the treatment of Addisonian anemia or Biermer's disease. III (with historical notes). Med. Rev. Rev. 38:487, 1932.
170. Gompertz, D. The metabolic effects of an impaired methylmalonyl CoA mutase. In The Cobalamins, Arnstein, H. R. V. and Wrighton, R. J., eds. Churchill Livingstone, Edinburgh, 1971, p. 101.
171. Goodman, J. R., Wallerstein, R. O., and Hall, S. G. The ultrastructure of bone marrow histiocytes in megaloblastic anaemia and the anaemia of infection. Brit. J. Haemat. 14:471, 1968.
172. Gottlieb, C. W., Retief, F. P., and Herbert, V. Blockade of vitamin B₁₂-binding sites in gastric juice, serum and saliva by analogues and derivatives of vitamin B₁₂ and by antibody to intrinsic factor. Biochim. Biophys. Acta 141:560, 1967.
173. Gowers, W. R. On the numeration of blood corpuscles. Lancet 2:797, 1877.
174. Graham, R. M. and Rheault, M. H. Characteristic cellular changes in epithelial cells in pernicious anemia. J. Lab. Clin. Med. 43:235, 1954.
175. Gräsbeck, R., Simons, K., and Sinkkonen, I. Isolation of intrinsic factor and its probable degradation product, as their vitamin B₁₂ complexes, from human gastric juice. Biochim. Biophys. Acta 127:47, 1966.

176. Gräsbeck, R. Intrinsic factor and the transcobalamins. Scand. J. Clin. Lab. Invest. Suppl. 95:7, 1967.

177. Greenfield, J. G., Blackwood, W., Meyer, A., McMenemey, W. H., and Norman, R. M. Neuropathology. Edward Arnold Publishers, Ltd., London, 1958.

178. Guest, J. R., Friedman, S., Woods, D. D., and Smith, E. L. A methyl analogue of cobamide coenzyme in relation to methionine synthesis by bacteria. Nature 195:340, 1962.

179. Guest, J. R., Foster, M. A., and Woods, D. D. Methyl derivatives of folic acid as intermediates in the methylation of homocysteine by Escherichia coli. Biochem. J. 92:488, 1964.

180. Hall, C. A. and Finkler, A. E. In vivo plasma vitamin B_{12} binding in B_{12} deficient and nondeficient subjects. J. Lab. Clin. Med. 60:765, 1962.

181. Hall, C. A. and Finkler, A. E. A second vitamin B_{12}-binding substance in human plasma. Biochim. Biophys. Acta 78:234, 1963.

182. Hall, C. A. and Finkler, A. E. The dynamics of transcobalamin II. A vitamin B_{12} binding substance in plasma. J. Lab. Clin. Med. 65;459, 1965.

183. Hall, C. A. and Finkler, A. E. Function of transcobalamin II. A B_{12} binding protein in human plasma. Proc. Soc. Exp. Biol. Med. 123:55, 1966.

184. Hall, C. A. and Finkler, A. E. Protein-mediated uptake of vitamin B_{12} by cells in tissue culture. In The Cobalamins, Arnstein, H. R. V. and Wrighton, R. J., eds. Churchill Livingstone, Edinburgh, 1971, p. 49.

185. Hall, M. Principles of the Theory and Practice of Medicine. Sherwood, Gilbert, and Piper, London, 1837.

186. Halsted, J. A., Gasster, M., and Drenick, E. J. Absorption of radioactive vitamin B_{12} after total gastrectomy. Relation to macrocytic anemia and to the site of origin of Castle's intrinsic factor. New Eng. J. Med. 251:161, 1954.

187. Hamilton, H. E., Sheets, R. F., and DeGowin, E. L. Studies with inagglutinable erythrocyte counts. VII. Further investigation of the hemolytic mechanism in untreated pernicious anemia and the demonstration of a hemolytic property in the plasma. J. Lab. Clin. Med. 51:942, 1958.

188. Hansky, J., Korman, M. G., Sovney, C., and St. John, D. J. B. Radioimmunoassay of gastrin: studies in pernicious anaemia. Gut 12:97, 1971.

189. Hardgrove, M., Yunck, R., Zotter, H., and Murphy, F. D. Summary of 80 living cases of pernicious anemia. Ann. Int. Med. 20:806, 1944.

190. Harker, L. A. and Finch, C. A. Thrombokinetics in man. J. Clin. Invest. 48:963, 1969.

191. Hatch, F. T., Larrabee, A. R., Cathou, R. E., and Buchanan, J. M. Enzymatic synthesis of the methyl group of methionine. I. Identification of the enzymes and cofactors involved in the system isolated from Escherichia coli. J. Biol. Chem. 236:1095, 1961.

192. Haurani, F. I., Sherwood, W., and Goldstein, F. Intestinal malabsorption of vitamin B_{12} in pernicious anemia. Metabolism 13:1342, 1964.

193. Hayem, G. and Nachet, A. Sur un nouveau procédé pour compter les globules du sang. Compt. Rend. l'Acad. Sci. 80:1083, 26 Avril 1875.

194. Hayem, G. Des degrés d'anémie. Bull. Mém. Soc. Mèd. Hosp. Paris 14:155, 1877.

195. Hayem, G. Des altérations anatomiques du sang dans l'anémie. Congrés Internat. des Sciences Med. 5me session, Genève, 9 au 15 Septembre 1877, p., 211.

196. Heath, C. W., Jr. Cytogenetic observations in vitamin B_{12} and folate deficiency. Blood 27:800, 1966.

197. Heinle, R. W. and Welch, A. D. Folic acid in pernicious anemia. Failure to prevent neurologic relapse. J. Amer. Med. Ass. 133:739, 1947.

198. Heinle, R. W., Welch, A. D., Scharf, V., Meacham, G. C., and Prusoff, W. H. Studies of excretion (and absorption) of Co 60-labeled vitamin B_{12} in pernicious anemia. Trans. Ass. Amer. Physicians 65:214, 1952.

199. Heller, P., West, M., and Zimmerman, H. J. Blood enzyme abnormalities in megaloblastic anemia. Clin. Res. 7:207, 1959.

200. Herbert, V. Studies on the role of intrinsic factor in vitamin B_{12} absorption, transport, and storage. Amer. J. Clin. Nutr. 7:433, 1959.

201. Herbert, V. and Zalusky, R. Interrelations of vitamin B_{12} and folic acid metabolism: folic acid clearance studies. J. Clin. Invest. 41:1263, 1962.

202. Herbert, V. and Castle, W. B. Intrinsic factor. New Eng. J. Med. 270:1181, 1964.

203. Herbert, V., Streiff, R. R., and Sullivan, L. W. Notes on vitamin B_{12} absorption, autoimmunity, and childhood pernicious anemia; relation of intrinsic factor to blood group substance. Medicine 43:679, 1964.

204. Herbert, V. and Sullivan, L. W. Activity of coenzyme B_{12} in man. Ann. N. Y. Acad. Sci. 112:855, 1964.

205. Herbert, V. Immunologic factors in pernicious anemia. Postgrad. Med. 42:298, 1967.

206. Herbert, V. Recent developments in cobalamin metabolism. In The Cobalamins, Arnstein, H. R. V. and Wrighton, R. J., eds. Churchill Livingstone, Edinburgh, 1971, p. 2.

207. Highley, D. R. and Ellenbogen, L. Studies on the mechanism of vitamin B_{12} absorption: in vivo transfer of vitamin B_{12} to intrinsic factor. Arch. Biochem. Biophys. 99:126, 1962.

208. Highley, D. R., Streiff, R. R., Ellenbogen, L., Herbert, V., and Castle, W. B. Releasing factor and endogenous vitamin B_{12}. Proc. Soc. Exp. Biol. Med. 119:565, 1965.

209. Hines, J. D., Rosenberg, A., and Harris, J. W. Intrinsic factor-mediated radio-B_{12} uptake in sequential incubation studies using everted sacs of guinea pig small intestine: evidence that intrinsic factor is not absorbed into the intestinal cell. Proc. Soc. Exp. Biol. Med. 129:653, 1968.

210. Hodgkin, D., Porter, M. W., and Spiller, R. C. Appendix. Crystallographic measurements on the anti-pernicious anaemia factor. Proc. Roy. Soc. Lond. Series B. 136:609, 1950.

211. Hodgkin, D. C., Pickworth, J., Robertson, J. H., Trueblood, K. N., Prosen, R. J., and White, J. G. The crystal structure of the hexacarboxylic acid derived from B_{12} and the molecular structure of the vitamin. Nature 176:325, 1955.

212. Hodgkin, D. C., Kamper, J., MacKay, M., Pickworth, J., Trueblood, K. N., and White, J. G. Structure of vitamin B_{12}. Nature 178:64, 1956.

213. Hoedemaeker, P. J., Abels, J., Wachters, J. J., Arends, A., and Nieweg, H. O. Further investigations about the site of production of Castle's gastric intrinsic factor. Lab. Invest. 15:1163, 1966.

214. Holmes, J. M. Cerebral manifestations of vitamin-B_{12} deficiency. Brit. Med. J. 2:1394, 1956.

215. Hooper, C. W. and Whipple, G. H. Blood regeneration after simple anaemia. I. Curve of regeneration influenced by dietary factors. Amer. J. Physiol. 45:573, 1918.

216. Horrigan, D., Jarrold, T., and Vilter, R. W. Direct action of vitamin B_{12} upon human bone marrow. J. Clin. Invest. 30:31, 1951.

217. Howard, R. P. Cases of pernicious progressive anaemia. Trans Inter. Med. Conf. Philadelphia, 1876, p. 432.

218. Hunter, W. Pernicious Anaemia. Charles Griffin and Co., Ltd. London, 1901.

219. Hunter, W. Severest Anaemias. Macmillan & Co., London, 1909.

220. Hurst, A. F. and Bell, J. R. The pathogenesis of subacute combined degeneration of the spinal cord, with special reference to its connection with Addison's (pernicious) anaemia, achlorhydria, and intestinal infection. Brain 45:266, 1922.

221. Hurst, A. F. An address on achlorhydria: its relation to pernicious anaemia and other diseases. Lancet 1:111, 1923.

222. Hutner, S. H., Provasoli, L., Stokstad, E. L. R., Hoffman, C. E., Belt, M., Franklin, A. L., and Jukes, T. H. Assay of anti-pernicious anemia factor with Euglena. Proc. Soc. Exp. Biol. Med. 70:118, 1949.

223. Irvine, W. J. Immunologic aspects of pernicious anemia. New Eng. J. Med. 273:432, 1965.

224. Isaacs, R. The leukocytes in pernicious anemia—physiology, pathology, and clinical significance. J. Clin. Invest. 6:28, 1928.

225. Isaacs, R. The erythrocytes. In Handbook of Hematology, Downey, H., ed. P. B. Hoeber, New York, Vol, 1, 1938, p. 25.

226. Jedlicka, V. Über die Lebertherapie und das Wesen der perniziösen Anämie. Folia Haemat. 42:359, 1930.

227. Jeffries, G. H. and Sleisenger, M. H. Studies of parietal cell antibody in pernicious anemia. J. Clin. Invest. 44:2021, 1965.

228. Jeffries, G. H., Todd, J. E., and Sleisenger, M. H. The effect of prednisolone on

gastric mucosal histology, gastric secretion, and vitamin B_{12} absorption in patients with pernicious anemia. J. Clin. Invest. 45:803, 1966.

229. Johns, D. G. and Bertino, J. R. Folates and megaloblastic anemia: A review. Clin. Pharmacol. Ther. 6:372, 1965.

230. Jones, O. P. Cytological studies of biopsied pernicious anemia bone marrow during relapse. Proc. Soc. Exp. Biol. Med. 34:694, 1936.

231. Jones, O. P. Cytology of pathologic marrow cells with special reference to bone-marrow biopsies. In Handbook of Hematology, Downey, H., ed. P. B. Hoeber, New York, 1938, vol. 3, p. 2043.

232. Jones, O. P. Morphologic, physiologic, chemical, and biologic distinction of megaloblasts. Arch. Path. 35:752, 1943.

233. Jones, O. P. The influence of disturbed metabolism on the morphology of blood cells. In Functions of the Blood, MacFarlane, R. G. and Robb-Smith, A. H. T., eds. Academic Press, New York, 1961, p. 171.

234. Kahler, O. and Pick, A. Über combinirte Systemerkrankungen des Rückenmarkes. Arch. Psychiat. 8:251, 1878.

235. Kampmeier, R. H. and Jones, E. Optic atrophy in pernicious anemia. Amer. J. Med. Sci. 195:633, 1938.

236. Kaplan, M. and Bernard, J. Maladie de Biermer chez une enfant de deux ans. Arch. Franc. Pediat. 3:161, 1946.

237. Kaplan, M. E., Zalusky, R., Remington, J., and Herbert, V. Immunologic studies with intrinsic factor in man. J. Clin. Invest. 42:368, 1963.

238. Kass, L. A clockface chromatin pattern in the intermediate megaloblast of vitamin B_{12} or folate deficiency. Blood 32:711, 1968.

239. Kass, L. Demonstration of histones in proerythroblasts in pernicious anemia and the DiGuglielmo syndrome. J. Histochem. Cytochem. 20:817, 1972.

240. Kass L. Histone biosynthesis in pernicious anemia proerythroblasts and megaloblasts. Blood 41:549, 1973.

241. Kass, L. Bone Marrow Interpretation. Charles C Thomas, Springfield, Ill., 1973.

242. Kass, L. Acetylation and methylation of histones in pernicious anemia. Blood 44:125, 1974.

243. Kass, L. Pink staining of pernicious anemia megaloblasts by alizarin red S. Amer. J. Clin. Path. 62:511, 1974.

244. Kass, L. and Schnitzer, B. Refractory Anemia. Charles C Thomas, Springfield, Ill., 1975.

245. Kass, L. and Gray, R. H. Ultrastructural localization of histones in chronic erythremic myelosis. Am. J. Path. 81:493, 1975.

246. Kass, L. Unusual morphologic abnormalities of megaloblasts in pernicious anemia and folate deficiency. Amer. J. Clin. Path. 65:177, 1976.

247. Kass, L. Origin and composition of Cabot rings in pernicious anemia. Amer. J. Clin. Path. 64:53, 1975.

248. Kass, L. and Hadi, M. Z. Phosphorylase activity in chronic erythremic myelosis. Amer. J. Clin. Path. 64:503, 1975.

249. Kaye, A. M. and Sheratzky, D. Methylation of protein (histone) in vitro: enzymic activity from the soluble fraction of rat organs. Biochim. Biophys. Acta 190:527, 1969.

250. Kellermeyer, R. W., Allen, S. H. G., Stjernholm, R., and Wood, H. G. Methylmalonyl isomerase IV. Purification and properties of the enzyme from propionibacteria. J. Biol. Chem. 239:2562, 1964.

251. Kelly, A. and Herbert, V. Coated charcoal assay of erythrocyte vitamin B_{12} levels. Blood 29:139, 1967.

252. Killander, D. and Rigler, R., Jr. Initial changes of deoxyribonucleoprotein and synthesis of nucleic acid in phytohemagglutinine-stimulated human leukocytes in vitro. Exp. Cell Res. 39:701, 1965.

253. Killmann, S. A. Effect of deoxyuridine on incorporation of tritiated thymidine: difference between normoblasts and megaloblasts. Acta Med. Scand. 175:483, 1964.

254. Kiossoglou, K. A., Mitus, W. J., and Dameshek, W. Chromosomal aberrations in pernicious anemia. Study of three cases before and after therapy. Blood 25:662, 1965.

255. Kristensen, H. P. Ø. and Friis, T. The mechanism of the prednisone effect upon B_{12} absorption in pernicious anaemia. Acta Med. Scand. *168*:457, 1960.

256. Kutzbach, C., Galloway, E., and Stokstad, E. L. R. Influence of vitamin B_{12} and methionine on levels of folic acid compounds and folate enzymes in rat liver. Proc. Soc. Exp. Biol. Med. *124*:801, 1967.

257. Laache, S. *Die Anämie*. Malling, Christiania (Oslo), 1883.

258. Lajtha, L. G. An inhibitory factor in pernicious anaemia serum. Clin. Sci. *9*:287, 1950.

259. Lajtha, L. G. Culture of human bone marrow *in vitro*. The reversibility between normoblastic and megaloblastic series of cells. J. Clin. Path. *5*:67, 1952.

260. Lajtha, L. G. and Kumatori, T. Nucleic acid metabolism in megaloblastic marrows *in vitro*. Nature *180*:991, 1957.

261. Lambert, H. P., Prankerd, T. A. J., and Smellie, J. M. Pernicious anaemia in childhood. Quart. J. Med. n.s. *30*:71, 1961.

262. Larrabee, A. R., Rosenthal, S., Cathou, R. E., and Buchanan, J. M. A methylated derivative of tetrahydrofolate as an intermediate of methionine synthesis. J. Amer. Chem. Soc. *83*:4094, 1961.

263. Larrabee, A. R., Rosenthal, S., Cathou, R. E., and Buchanan, J. M. Enzymatic synthesis of the methyl group of methionine. IV. Isolation, characterization and role of 5-methyltetrahydrofolate. J. Biol. Chem. *238*:1025, 1963.

264. Latner, A. L. Intrinsic factor and vitamin B_{12} absorption. Brit. Med. J. *2*:278, 1958.

265. Lazarus, A. Progressive pernicious anemia. In *Diseases of the Blood*, Stengel, A., ed. W. B. Saunders, Philadelphia, 1905, p. 227.

266. Lear, A., Harris, J. W., Castle, W. B., and Fleming, E. M. The serum vitamin concentration in pernicious anemia. J. Lab. Clin. Med. *44*:715, 1954.

267. Lee, R. I., Minot, G. R., and Vincent, B. Splenectomy in pernicious aner Studies on bone marrow stimulation. J. Amer. Med. Ass. *67*:719, 1916.

268. Leichtenstern, O. Ueber progressive perniciöse Anämie bei Tabeskranken. Deutsch. Med. Wschr. *10*:849, 1884.

269. Lengyel, P., Mazumder, R., and Ochoa, S. Mammalian methylmalonyl isomerase and vitamin B_{12} coenzymes. Proc. Nat. Acad. Sci. *46*:1312, 1960.

270. Lerman, J. and Means, J. H. The gastric secretion in exophthalmic goitre and myxoedema. J. Clin. Invest. *11*:167, 1932.

271. Lessin, L. S. and Bessis, M. Morphology of the erythron. In *Hematology*. Williams, W. J. et al., eds. McGraw-Hill, New York, 1972, p. 77.

272. Lessner, H. E. and Friedkin, M. The *in vitro* incorporation of deoxyuridine and thymidine into the deoxyribonucleic acid of human megaloblastic and normoblastic bone marrows. Clin. Res. *7*:207, 1959.

273. Levine, S. A. and Ladd, W. S. Pernicious anemia. A clinical study of one hundred and fifty consecutive cases with special reference to gastric anacidity. Johns Hopkins Hosp. Bull. *32*:254, 1921.

274. Lichtheim, L. Zur Kenntniss der perniziösen Anämie. München. Med. Wschr. *34*:300, 1887.

275. Liu, Y. K. and Sullivan, L. W. Marrow granulocyte reserve in pernicious anemia. Clin. Res. (abstract) *14*:321, 1966.

276. Lloyd, J. H. The spinal cord in pernicious anaemia. J. Nerv. Ment. Dis. n.s. *21*:225, 1896.

277. London, I. M. and West, R. The formation of bile pigment in pernicious anemia. J. Biol. Chem. *184*:359, 1950.

278. Loughlin, R. E., Elford, H. L, and Buchanan, J. M. Enzymatic synthesis of the methyl group of methionine. VII. Isolation of a cobalamin-containing transmethylase (5-methyltetrahydrofolate-homocysteine) from mammalian liver. J. Biol. Chem. *239*:2888, 1964.

279. Lous, P. and Schwartz, M. The absorption of vitamin B_{12} following partial gastrectomy. Acta Med. Scand. *164*:407, 1959.

280. Lynch, E. C. and Alfrey, C. P., Jr. Studies *in vitro* on the autohemolysis of normoblastic and megaloblastic marrow cells. Tex. Rep. Biol. Med. *24*:180, 1966.

281. MacDonald, R. M., Ingelfinger, F. J., and Belding, H. W. Late effects of total gastrectomy in man. New Eng. J. Med. *237*:887, 1947.

282. MacKenzie, S. Clinical lecture on idiopathic, essential, or progressive pernicious anemia. Lancet *2*:797, 833, 1878.

283. Martin, C. J. Diseases of stock in Australia caused by deficiency of cobalt and of both cobalt and copper. Proc. Nutr. Soc. *1*:195, 1944.

284. Massey, B. W. and Rubin, C. E. The stomach in pernicious anemia: a cytologic study. Amer. J. Med. Sci. *227*:481, 1954.

285. McGuigan, J. E. Measurement of the affinity of human gastric intrinsic factor for cyanocobalamin. J. Lab. Clin. Med. *70*:666, 1967.

286. McIntyre, O. R., Sullivan, L. W., Jeffries, G. H., and Silver, R. H. Pernicious anemia in childhood. New Eng. J. Med. *272*:981, 1965.

287. McIntyre, P. A., Hahn, R., Conley, C. L., and Glass, B. Genetic factors in predisposition to pernicious anemia. Bull. Johns Hopkins Hosp. *104*:309,1959.

288. McIntyre, P. A. Genetic and auto-immune features of pernicious anemia. I. Unreliability of the Schilling test in detecting genetic predisposition to the disease. Johns Hopkins Med. J. *122*:181, 1968.

289. Mendelsohn, R. S., Watkin, D. M., Horbett, A. P., and Fahey, J. L. Identification of the vitamin B_{12}–binding protein in the serum of normals and of patients with chronic myelocytic leukemia. Blood *13*:740, 1958.

290. Menzies, R. C., Crossen, P. E., Fitzgerald, P. H., and Gunz, F. W. Cytogenetic and cytochemical studies on marrow cells in B_{12} and folate deficiency. Blood *28*:581, 1966.

291. Messner, H., Fliedner, T. M., and Cronkite, E. P. Kinetics of erythropoietic cell proliferation in pernicious anemia. Ser. Haemat. n.s. *2(4)*:44, 1969.

292. Metz, J., Kelly, A., Swett, V. C., Waxman, S., and Herbert, V. Deranged DNA synthesis by bone marrow from vitamin B_{12}–deficient humans. Brit. J. Haemat. *14*:575, 1968.

293. Miller, A. and Sullivan, J. F. The *in vitro* binding of Co60 labeled vitamin B_{12} by normal and leukemic sera. J. Clin. Invest. *37*:556, 1958.

294. Miller, A. and Sullivan, J. F. Electrophoretic studies of the vitamin B_{12}–binding protein of normal and chronic myelogenous leukemia serum. J. Clin. Invest. *38*:2135, 1959.

295. Minnich, W. Zur Kenntniss der im Verlaufe der perniziösen Anämie beobachteten Spinalerkrankungen. Z. Klin. Med. *21*:25, 260, 1893 and *22*:60, 1893.

296. Minot, G. R. Two curable cases of anemia. Med. Clin. N. Amer. *4*:1733, 1921.

297. Minot, G. R. and Murphy, W. P. Observations on patients with pernicious anemia partaking of a special diet. A. Clinical aspects. Murphy, W. P., Fitz, R., and Monroe, R. D. B. Physiological aspects. Trans. Assoc. Amer. Phys. *41*:72, 1926.

298. Minot, G.R. and Murphy, W. P. Treatment of pernicious anemia by a special diet. J. Amer. Med. Ass. *87*:470, 1926.

299. Minot, G. R. and Castle, W. B. The interpretation of reticulocyte reactions. Their value in determining the potency of therapeutic materials, especially in pernicious anemia. Lancet *2*:319, 1935.

300. Minot, G. R. The development of liver therapy in pernicious anemia. In *Les Prix Nobel en 1934*. Norstedt, Stockholm, 1935.

301. Möller, (initial unavailable). Klinische Bemerkungen über einige weniger bekannte Krankheiten der Zunge. Deutsch. Klin. *3*:273, 1851.

302. Moyer, A. W. and du Vigneaud, V. The structural specificity of choline and betaine in transmethylation. J. Biol. Chem. *143*:373, 1942.

303. Murphy, W. P. and Minot, G. R. A special diet for patients with pernicious anemia. Boston Med. Surg. J. *195*:410, 1926.

304. Murphy, W. P. Pernicious anemia. In *Les Prix Nobel en 1934*. Norstedt, Stockholm, 1935.

305. Murphy, W. P. *Anemia in Practice. Pernicious Anemia*. W. B. Saunders, Philadelphia, 1939.

306. Murphy, W. P. and Whipple, G. H. as quoted in Medicine's Living History: Recollections of liver therapy. Medical World News. *13*(33):37, Sept. 8, 1972 (quoted with permission of Medical World News).

307. Myhre, E. Studies on megaloblasts *in vitro*. I. Proliferation and destruction of nucleated red cells in pernicious anemia before and during treatment with vitamin B_{12}. Scand. J. Clin. Lab. Invest. *16*:307, 1964.

308. Myhre, E. Studies on megaloblasts *in vitro*. II. Maturation of nucleated red cells in pernicious anemia before and during treatment with vitamin B_{12}. Scand. J. Clin. Lab. Invest. *16*:320, 1964.

309. Nathan, D. G. and Gardner, F. H. Erythroid cell maturation and hemoglobin synthesis in megaloblastic anemia. J. Clin. Invest. 41:1086, 1962.

310. Neumann, E. Ueber die Bedeutung des Knochenmarks für die Blutbildung. Centralbl. Med. Wissensch. 6:689, 1868.

311. Nixon, P. F. and Bertino, J. R. Interrelationships of vitamin B_{12} and folate in man. Amer. J. Med. 48:555, 1970.

312. Nixon, P. F. and Bertino, J. R. Impaired utilization of serum folate in pernicious anemia. A study with radiolabeled 5-methyltetrahydrofolate. J. Clin. Invest. 51:1431, 1972.

313. Noronha, J. M. and Silverman, M. On folic acid, vitamin B_{12}, methionine, and formiminoglutamic acid metabolism. *Vitamin B_{12} and intrinsic factor. Second European Symposium*, Heinrich, H. C., ed. Hamburg, 1961. Ferdinand Enke Verlag, Stuttgart, 1962.

314. Okuda, K. and Fujii, T. *In vitro* digestion of intrinsic factor-vitamin B_{12} complex and release of vitamin B_{12}. Arch. Biochem. Biophys. 115:302, 1966.

315. Osler, W. and Gardner, W. Ueber die Beschaffenheit des Blutes und Knochenmarkes in der progressiven perniciösen Anämie. Centralbl. Med. Wissensch. 15:258, 1877.

316. Osler, W. Beschaffenheit des Blutes und Knochemarkes bei perniciöser Anämie. Centralbl. Med. Wissensch. 15:498, 1877.

317. Paik, W. K. and Kim, S. Protein methylation. Science 174:114, 1971.

318. Pant, S. S., Asbury, A. K., and Richardson, E. P. The myelopathy of pernicious anemia. A neuropathological reappraisal. Acta Neurol. Scand. Suppl. 35, 1968.

319. Paranchych, W. and Cooper, B. A. Factors influencing the uptake of cyanocobalamin (vitamin B_{12}) by Ehrlich ascites carcinoma cells. Biochim. Biophys. Acta 60:393, 1962.

320. Peabody, F. W. and Broun, G. O. Phagocytosis by erythrocytes in the bone marrow with special reference to pernicious anemia. Amer. J. Path. 1:169, 1925.

321. Peabody, F. W. The pathology of the bone marrow in pernicious anemia. Amer. J. Path. 3:179, 1927.

322. Pedersen, J., Lund, J., Ohlsen, A. S., and Kristensen, H. P. Ø. Partial megaloblastic erythropoiesis in elderly achlorhydric patients with mild anaemia. Lancet 1:448, 1957.

323. Pepper, O. H. P. and Peet, M. M. The resistance of reticulated erythrocytes. Arch. Int. Med. 12:81, 1913.

324. Pepper, W. Progressive pernicious anaemia, or anaematosis. Amer. J. Med. Sci. n.s. 70:313, 1875.

325. Perillie, P. E., Kaplan, S. S., and Finch, S. C. Significance of changes in serum muramidase activity in megaloblastic anemia. New Eng. J. Med. 277:10, 1967.

326. Peters, T. J. and Hoffbrand, A. V. Absorption of vitamin B_{12} by the guinea-pig: The role of the ileal mitochondrion. In *The Cobalamins*, Arnstein, H. R. V. and Wrighton, R. J., eds. Churchill Livingstone, Edinburgh, 1971, p. 61.

327. Peterson, J. C. and Dunn, S. C. Pernicious anemia in childhood. Amer. J. Dis. Child. 71:252, 1946.

328. Pitney, W. R., Beard, M. F., and Van Loon, E. J. Observations on the bound form of vitamin B_{12} in human serum. J. Biol. Chem. 207:143, 1954.

329. Pogo, B. G. T., Allfrey, V. G., and Mirsky, A. E. RNA synthesis and histone acetylation during the course of gene activation in lymphocytes. Proc. Nat. Acad. Sci. 55:805, 1966.

330. Pohl, C. Über perniziöse Anämie im Kindesalter. Mschr. Kind. 84:192, 1940.

331. Powsner, E. R. and Berman, L. Human bone marrow chromosomes in megaloblastic anemia. Blood 26:784, 1965.

332. Pratt, J. M. *Inorganic Chemistry of Vitamin B_{12}*. Academic Press, London, 1972.

333. Preyer, W. *Die Blutkrystalle*. Mauke, Jena, 1871.

334. Putnam, J. J. A group of cases of system scleroses of the spinal cord, associated with diffuse collateral degeneration; occurring in enfeebled persons past middle life, and especially in women; studied with particular reference to etiology. J. Nerv. Ment. Dis. 18:69, 1891.

335. Putnam, J. J. Cases of myxoedema and acromegalia treated with benefit by sheep's thyroids. Trans. Ass. Amer. Physicians 8:333, 1893.

336. Putnam, J. J. and Taylor, E. W. Diffuse degeneration of the spinal cord. J. Nerv. Ment. Dis. 28:74, 1901.

337. Pye-Smith, P. H. Idiopathic anaemia of Addison. Guy's Hosp. Report 41:219, 1882.

338. Quincke, H. A lecture on pernicious anaemia. Med. Times Gaz. 2:374, 428, 1876.

339. Quincke, H. Über perniziöse Anämie. Centralbl. Med. Wissensch. 15:849, 1877.

340. Quincke, H. Weitere Beobachtungen über perniziöse Anämie. Deutsch Arch. Klin. Med. 20:1, 1877.

341. Reisner, E. H., Wolff, J. A., McKay, J., and Doyle, E. F. Juvenile pernicious anemia. Pediatrics 8:88, 1951.

342. Reisner, E. H. and Korson, R. Microspectrophotometric determination of deoxyribosenucleic acid in megaloblasts of pernicious anemia. Blood 6:344, 1961.

343. Retey, J. and Arigoni, D. Coenzym B_{12} als gemeinsamer Wasserstoffüberträger der Dioldehydrase und der Methylmalonyl-CoA-Mutase-Reaktion. Experientia 22:783, 1966.

344. Retief, F. P., Gottlieb, C. W., and Herbert, V. Mechanisms of vitamin B_{12} uptake by erythrocytes. J. Clin. Invest. 45:1907, 1966.

345. Rickes, E. L., Brink, N. G., Koniuszy, F. R., Wood, T. R., and Folkers, K. Crystalline vitamin B_{12}. Science 107:396, 1948.

346. Rickes, E. L., Brink, N. G., Koniuszy, F. R., Wood, T. R., and Folkers, K. Comparative data on vitamin B_{12} from liver and from a new source, Streptomyces griseus. Science 108:634, 1948.

347. Riggs, C. E. Some nervous symptoms of pernicious anemia. J. Amer. Med. Ass. 61:481, 1913.

348. Robbins, E. and Borun, T. W. The cytoplasmic synthesis of histones in HeLa cells and its temporal relationship to DNA replication. Proc. Nat. Acad. Sci. U.S.A. 57:409 1967.

349. Robscheit-Robbins, F. S. and Whipple, G. H. Blood regeneration in severe anemia. II. Favorable influence of liver, heart and skeletal muscle in diet. Amer. J. Physiol. 72:408, 1925.

350. Rondanelli, E. G., Gorini, P., Magliulo, E., and Fiori, G. P. Differences in proliferative activity between normoblasts and pernicious anemia megaloblasts. Blood 24:542, 1964.

351. Rosenblum, C. and Woodbury, D. T. Cobalt 60 labeled vitamin B_{12} of high specific activity. Science 113:215, 1951.

352. Ross, G. I. M. Vitamin B_{12} assay in body fluids. Nature 166:270, 1950.

353. Ross, G. I. M. Vitamin B_{12} assay in body fluids using Euglena gracilis. J. Clin. Path. 5:250, 1952.

354. Rothenberg, S. P. and Huhti, A. L. Identification of a macromolecular factor in the ileum which binds intrinsic factor and immunologic identification of intrinsic factor in ileal extracts. J. Clin. Invest. 47:913, 1968.

355. Rosenszajn, L., Leibovich, M., Shoham, D., and Epstein, J. The esterase activity in megaloblasts, leukaemic and normal haematopoietic cells. Brit. J. Haemat. 14:605, 1968.

356. Rous, P. Urinary siderosis. Hemosiderin granules in the urine as an aid in the diagnosis of pernicious anemia, hemochromatosis, and other diseases causing siderosis of the kidney. J. Exp. Med. 28:645, 1918.

357. Russell, J. S. R. The relationship of some forms of combined degenerations of the spinal cord to one another and to anaemia. Lancet 2:4, 1898.

358. Russell, J. S. R., Batten, F. E., and Collier, J. Subacute combined degeneration of the spinal cord. Brain 23:39, 1900.

359. Saltzman, F. Bothriocephalus, liver-therapy, and reticulocyte-reaction. Acta Med. Scand. Suppl. 34:75, 1930.

360. Samloff, I. M., Kleinman, M. S., Turner, M. D., Sobel, M. V., and Jeffries, G. H. Blocking and binding antibodies to intrinsic factor and parietal cell antibody in pernicious anemia. Gastroenterology 55:575, 1968.

361. Sauli, S., Astaldi, G., and Malossini, L. Histopathology of intestinal mucosa obtained by Crosby's biopsy in pernicious anemia before and after vitamin B_{12} treatment. Acta Vitamin. (Milano) 17:143, 1963.

362. Schade, S. G., Feick, P. L., Muckerheide, M., and Schilling, R. F. Occurrence in gastric juice of antibody to a complex of intrinsic factor and vitamin B_{12}. New Eng. J. Med. 275:528, 1966.

363. Schade, S. G., Feick, P. L., Imrie, M. H., and Schilling, R. F. *In vitro* studies on antibodies to intrinsic factor. Clin. Exp. Immun. 2:399, 1967.

364. Schilling, R. F. Intrinsic factor studies. II. The effect of gastric juice on the urinary excretion of radioactivity after the oral administration of radioactive vitamin B_{12}. J. Lab. Clin. Med. 42:860, 1953.

365. Schleicher, E. M. Giant orthochromatic erythroblasts. Their importance for the promegaloblast and pronormoblast problem. J. Lab. Clin. Med. 29:127, 1944.

366. Schloesser, L. L. and Schilling, R. F. Vitamin B_{12} absorption studies in a vegetarian with megaloblastic anemia. Amer. J. Clin. Nutr. 12:70, 1963.

367. Schnitzer, B., Aikawa, M., and Spencer, H. H. Pernicious anemia. An ultrastructural study of the bone marrow before and after vitamin B_{12} therapy. Amer. J. Clin. Path. 58:1, 1972.

368. Schwartz, M. Intrinsic-factor-inhibiting substance in serum of orally treated patients with pernicious anemia. Lancet 2:61, 1958.

369. Schwarz, E. Cellular gigantism and pluripolar mitosis in human hematopoiesis. Amer. J. Anat. 79:75, 1946.

370. Shorb, M. S. Unidentified growth factors for *Lactobacillus lactis* in refined liver extracts. J. Biol. Chem. 169:455, 1947.

371. Shorb, M. S. Activity of vitamin B_{12} for the growth of *Lactobacillus lactis*. Science 107:397, 1948.

372. Silber, R., Fujioka, S., Moldow, C. F., and Cox, R. Altered regulation of deoxyribonucleotide synthesis in B_{12} or folate deficiency. Clin. Res. 18:416, 1970.

373. Silber, R. and Moldow, C. F. The biochemistry of B_{12}-mediated reactions in man. Amer. J. Med. 48:549, 1970.

374. Smith, A. D. M. Megaloblastic madness. Brit. Med. J. 2:1840, 1960.

375. Smith, E. L. Purification of anti-pernicious anaemia factors from liver. Nature 161:638, 1948.

376. Smith, E. L. and Parker, L. F. J. Purification of antipernicious anaemia factor. Biochem. J. 43:VIII, 1948.

377. Smith, E. L. Presence of cobalt in the anti-pernicious anaemia factor. Nature 162:144, 1948.

378. Smith, T. On changes in the red blood-corpuscles in the pernicious anaemia of Texas cattle fever. Trans. Ass. Amer. Physicians 6:263, 1891.

379. Spies, T. D. and Stone, R. E. Liver extract, folic acid, and thymine in pernicious anaemia and subacute combined degeneration. Lancet 1:174, 1947.

380. Spies, T. D., Frommeyer, W. B., Jr., Vilter, C. F., and English, A. Anti-anemic properties of thymine. Blood 1:185, 1946.

381. Spray, G. H. and Witts, L. J. Thymidine in megaloblastic anaemia. Lancet 2:869, 1958.

382. Stokstad, E. L. R., Page, A., Jr., Pierce, J., Franklin, A. L., Jukes, T. H., Heinle, R. W., Epstein, M., and Welch, A. D. Activity of microbial animal protein factor concentrates in pernicious anemia. J. Lab. Clin. Med. 33:860, 1948.

383. Strauss, E. W. and Wilson, T. H. Factors controlling B_{12} uptake by intestinal sacs *in vitro*. Amer. J. Physiol. 198:103, 1960.

384. Strauss, M. B. Of medicine, men and molecules: Wedlock or divorce. Medicine 43:619, 1964.

385. Stuart, J. and Skowron, P. N. A cytochemical study of marrow enzymes in megaloblastic anaemia. Brit. J. Haemat. 15:443, 1968.

386. Sturgis, C. C. and Isaacs, R. Desiccated stomach in the treatment of pernicious anemia. J. Amer. Med. Ass. 93:747, 1929.

387. Sturgis, C. C. *Hematology* (First edition). Charles C Thomas, Springfield, Ill. 1948.

388. Sullivan, L. W. and Herbert, V. Studies on the minimum daily requirement for vitamin B_{12}. New Eng. J. Med. 272:340, 1965.

389. Sullivan, L. W., Herbert, V., and Castle, W. B. *In vitro* assay for human intrinsic factor. J. Clin. Invest. 42:1443, 1963.

390. Tabor, H., Silverman, M., Mehler, A. H., Daft, F. S., and Bauer, H. L-histidine conversion to a urinary glutamic acid derivative in folic-deficient rats. J. Amer. Chem. Soc. 75:756, 1953.

391. Tai, C. and McGuigan, J. E. Immunologic studies in pernicious anemia. Blood
     34:63, 1969.
392. Takeyama, S., Hatch, F. T., and Buchanan, J. M. Enzymatic synthesis of the
     methyl group of methionine. II. Involvement of vitamin B_{12}. J. Biol. Chem.
     236:1102, 1961.
393. Taylor, K. B. Inhibition of intrinsic factor by pernicious anaemia sera. Lancet
     2:106, 1959.
394. Taylor, R. T. and Weissbach, H. N^5-methyltetrahydrofolate-homocysteine trans-
     methylase. Role of S-adenosylmethionine in vitamin B_{12}-dependent methionine
     synthesis. J. Biol. Chem. 242:1517, 1967.
395. Taylor, R. T. and Weissbach, H. *Escherichia coli B* N^5-methyltetrahydrofolate-
     homocysteine vitamin B_{12} transmethylase: formation and photolability of a
     methylcobalamin enzyme. Arch. Biochem. Biophys. 123:109, 1968.
396. Taylor, R.T., Hanna, M. L., and Hutton, J. J. 5-Methyltetrahydrofolate homocys-
     teine cobalamin methyltransferase in human bone marrow and its relationship
     to pernicious anemia. Arch. Biochem. Biophys. 165:787, 1974.
397. Tempka, T. and Braun, B. Das morphologische Verhalten des Sternumpunktates
     in verschiedenen Stadien der perniziösen Anämie und seine Wandlungen unter
     dem Einflusse der Therapie. Folia Haemat. 48:355, 1932.
398. Thomas, E. D. and Lochte, H. L. Studies on the biochemical defect of pernicious
     anemia. I. In vitro observations on oxygen consumption, heme synthesis, and
     deoxyribonucleic acid synthesis by pernicious anemia bone marrow. J. Clin.
     Invest. 37:166, 1958.
399. Thompson, R. B. Addisonian pernicious anaemia. Confirmatory evidence of a fac-
     tor inhibiting erythropoiesis. Clin. Sci. 9:281, 1950.
400. Thompson, R. B. Observations on the effects of vitamin B_{12}, liver extracts, folic
     acid, and thymine on the maturation of megaloblasts in culture. Blood 7:522,
     1952.
401. Thorn, G. W., Forsham, P. H., Frawley, T. F., Hill, S. R., Jr., Roche, M., Staehelin,
     D., and Wilson, D. L. The clinical usefulness of ACTH and cortisone (con-
     cluded). New Eng. J. Med. 242:865, 1950.
402. Tidwell, T., Allfrey, V. G., and Mirsky, A. E. The methylation of histones during
     regeneration of the liver. J. Biol. Chem. 243:707, 1968.
403. Toohey, J. I. and Barker, H. A. Isolation of coenzyme B_{12} from liver. J. Biol. Chem.
     236:560, 1961.
404. Tsamboulas, N. and Malikiosis, X. Zur Frage der Cabotschen Ringkörper.
     Deutsch. Arch. Klin. Med. 184:183, 1939.
405. Tudhope, G. R. and Wilson, G. M. Anaemia in hypothyroidism. Quart. J. Med.
     53(n.s. 29):513, 1960.
406. Tudhope, G. R. and Wilson, G. M. Deficiency of vitamin B_{12} in hypothyroidism.
     Lancet 1:703, 1962.
407. Van der Scheer, W. M. and Koek, H. C. Peripheral nerve lesions in cases of
     pernicious anaemia. Acta Psych. Neurol. 13:61, 1938.
408. Van der Weyden, M., Rother, M., and Firkin, B. Megaloblastic maturation masked
     by iron deficiency: a biochemical basis. Brit. J. Haemat. 22:299, 1972.
409. Vierordt, K. Neue Methode der quantitativen mikroskopischen. Analyse des
     Blutes. Arch. Phys. Heilk. 11:26, 1852.
410. Vilter, R. W., Horrigan, D., Mueller, J. F., Jarrold, T., Vilter, C. F., Hawkin, V., and
     Seaman, A. Studies on the relationships of vitamin B_{12}, folic acid, thymine,
     uracil, and methyl group donors in persons with pernicious anemia and related
     megaloblastic anemias. Blood 5:695, 1950.
411. Vivacqua, R. J., Myerson, R. M., Prescott, D. J., and Rabinowitz, J. L. Abnormal
     propionic-methylmalonic-succinic acid metabolism in vitamin B_{12} deficiency
     and its possible relationship to the neurologic syndrome of pernicious anemia.
     Amer. J. Med. Sci. 251:507, 1966.
412. Waife, S. O., Jansen, C. J., Crabtree, R. E., Grinnan, E. L., and Fouts, P. J. Oral
     vitamin B_{12} without intrinsic factor in the treatment of pernicious anemia. Ann.
     Int. Med. 58:810, 1963.
413. Wallerstein, R. O. and Pollycove, M. Bone marrow hemosiderin and ferrokinetics
     patterns in anemia. II. Pernicious anemia. Arch. Int. Med. 101:418, 1958.
414. Warthin, A. S. The pathology of pernicious anaemia, with special reference to
     changes occurring in the haemolymph nodes (eight autopsy cases). Amer. J.
     Med. Sci. 124:674, 1902.

415. Waxman, S., Metz, J., and Herbert, V. Defective DNA synthesis in human megaloblastic bone marrow: effects of homocysteine and methionine. J. Clin. Invest.
48:284, 1969.
416. Waxman, S., Corcino, J. J., and Herbert, V. Drugs, toxins, and dietary amino acids
affecting vitamin B_{12} or folic acid absorption or utilization. Amer. J. Med.
48:599, 1970.
417. Wearn, J. T., Warren, S., and Ames, O. The length of life of transfused erythrocytes
in patients with primary and secondary anemia. Arch. Int. Med. 29:527, 1922.
418. Weil, A. and Davison, C. Changes in the spinal cord in anemia. A clinicomicro-
scopic study. Arch. Neurol. Psych. 22:966, 1929.
419. Weinstein, I. B., Weissman, S. M., and Watkin, D. M. The plasma vitamin B_{12}
binding substance. I. Its detection in the seromucoid fraction of plasma from
normal subjects and patients with chronic myelocytic leukemia. J. Clin. Invest.
38:1904, 1959.
420. Weisberg. H., Rhodin, J., and Glass, G. B. J. Intestinal vitamin B_{12} absorption in
the dog. III. Demonstration of the intracellular pathway of absorption by light
and electron microscope autoradiography. Lab. Invest. 19:516, 1968.
421. Weissbach, H., Redfield, B. G., and Dickerman, H. Effect of vitamin B_{12} analogues
on methionine formation from N^5 methyltetrahydrofolic acid. J. Biol. Chem.
239:146, 1964.
422. Weissbach, H. and Taylor, R. T. Metabolic role of vitamin B_{12}. Vitam. Horm.
26:395, 1968.
423. West, R. Activity of vitamin B_{12} in Addisonian pernicious anemia. Science 107:398,
1948.
424. Whipple, G. H., Robscheit, F. S., and Hooper, C. W. Blood regeneration following
simple anemia. IV. Influence of meat, liver, and various extractives, alone or
combined with standard diets. Amer. J. Physiol. 53:236, 1920.
425. Whipple, G. H. Pigment metabolism and regeneration of hemoglobin in the body.
Arch. Int. Med. 29:711, 1922.
426. Whipple, G. H. and Robscheit-Robbins, F. S. Blood regeneration in severe
anemia. I. Standard basal ration bread and experimental methods. Amer. J.
Physiol. 72:395, 1925.
427. Whipple, G. H. and Robscheit-Robbins, F. S. Blood regeneration in severe
anemia. III. Iron reaction favorable-arsenic and germanium dioxide almost inert. Amer. J. Physiol. 72:419, 1925.
428. Whipple, G. H. Hemoglobin regeneration as influenced by diet and other factors.
In Les Prix Nobel en 1934. Norstedt, Stockholm, 1935.
429. White, J. C., Leslie, I., and Davidson, J. N. Nucleic acids of bone marrow cells,
with special reference to pernicious anemia. J. Path. Bact. 66:291, 1953.
430. Whittingham, S., Ungar, B., Mackay, I. R., and Mathews, J. D. The genetic factor in
pernicious anaemia. A family study in patients with gastritis. Lancet 1:951,
1969.
431. Wickramasinghe, S. N., Chalmers, D. G., and Cooper, E. H. Disturbed proliferation of erythropoietic cells in pernicious anaemia. Nature 215:189, 1967.
432. Wickramasinghe, S. N., Cooper, E. H., and Chalmers, D. G. A study of erythropoiesis by combined morphologic, quantitative cytochemical and autoradiographic methods. Blood 31:304, 1968.
433. Wickramasinghe, S. N., Chalmers, D. G., and Cooper, E. H. Arrest of cell proliferation and protein synthesis in megaloblasts of pernicious anemia. Acta Haemat.
41:65, 1969.
434. Wickramasinghe, S. N. and Pratt, J. R. Myelocyte proliferation in pernicious
anaemia. Acta Haemat. 44:37, 1970.
435. Wickramasinghe, S. N. and Longland, J. E. Rate of incorporation of tritiated
thymidine into DNA of normoblastic and megaloblastic bone marrow cells in
vitro. Acta Haemat. 52:14, 1974.
436. Williams, A. M., Chosy, J. J., and Schilling, R. F. Effect of vitamin B_{12} in vitro on
incorporation of nucleic acid precursors by pernicious anemia bone marrow. J.
Clin. Invest. 42:670, 1963.
437. Wills, L. and Evans, B. D. F. Tropical macrocytic anaemia. Its relation to pernicious anaemia. Lancet 2:416, 1938.

438. Wintrobe, M. M. The antianemic effect of yeast in pernicious anemia. Amer. J. Med. Sci. 197:286, 1939.
439. Wintrobe, M. M., Cartwright, G. E., Palmer, J. G., Kuhns, W. J., and Samuels, L. T. Effects of corticotrophin and cortisone on the blood in various disorders in man. Arch. Int. Med. 88:310, 1951.
440. Woltman, H. W. Brain changes associated with pernicious anemia. Arch. Int. Med. 21:791, 1918.
441. Wood, H. G., Kellermeyer, R. W., Stjernholm, R., and Allen, S. H. G. Metabolism of methylmalonyl CoA and the role of biotin and B_{12}-coenzymes. Ann. N.Y. Acad. Sci. 112:661, 1964.
442. Woodward, R. B. The total synthesis of vitamin B_{12}. Pure Appl. Chem. 33:145, 1973 (given Feb. 12, 1972).
443. Yates, T. and Cooper, B. A. Failure to demonstrate that antibody to intrinsic factor is a significant cause of vitamin B_{12} malabsorption in pernicious anemia. Canad. Med. Ass. J. 97:950, 1967.
444. Yoshida, Y., Todo, A., Shirakawa, S., Wakisaka, G., and Uchino, H. Proliferation of megaloblasts in pernicious anemia as observed from nucleic acid metabolism. Blood 31:292, 1968.
445. Zalusky, R. and Herbert, V. Failure of formiminoglutamic acid (FiGlu) excretion to distinguish vitamin B_{12} deficiency from nutritional folic acid deficiency. J. Clin. Invest. (abstract) 40:1091, 1961.
446. Zarafonetis, C. J. D., Overman, R. L., and Molthan, L. Unique sequence of pernicious anemia, polycythemia, and acute leukemia. Blood 12:1011, 1957.

INDEX

Page numbers in *italics* refer to figures; page numbers followed by (t) refer to tables.

239

MAJOR PROBLEMS IN INTERNAL MEDICINE

Cline: Cancer Chemotherapy (Second Edition, by Cline and Haskell, now available separately from the publisher)
Shearn: Sjögren's Syndrome
Cogan: Opthalmic Manifestations of Systemic Vascular Disease
Williams:Rheumatoid Arthritis as a Systemic Disease
Cluff, Caranasos and Stewart: Clinical Problems with Drugs
Fries and Holman: Systemic Lupus Erythematosus

In Preparation

Braude: Antimicrobial Drug Therapy
Bray: The Obese Patient
Gorlin: Coronary Artery Disease
Ingbar: Pathophysiology and Diagnosis of Disorders of the Thyroid
Krugman and Ward: Viral Hepatitis
Potts: Disorders of Calcium Metabolism
Felig: Diabetes Mellitus
Bunn, Forget and Ranney: Normal and Abnormal Hemoglobins
Sleisenger: Malabsorption
Havel and Kane: Diagnosis and Treatment of Hyperlipidemias
Siltzbach: Sarcoidosis
Scheinberg and Sternlieb: Wilson's Disease and Copper Metabolism
Atkins and Bodel: Fever
Lieber and De Carli: Medical Aspects of Alcoholism
Merrill: Glomerulonephritis
Goldberg: The Scientific Basis and Practical Use of Diuretics
Laragh; Reversible Hypertension
Kilbourne: Influenza
Deykin: Diseases of the Platelets
Schwartz and Lergier: Immunosuppressive Therapy
Cohen: Amyloidosis
Seegmiller: Gout
Weinstein: Infective Endocarditis
Sasahara: Pulmonary Embolism
Zieve and Levin: Disorders of Hemostasis
Smith: Renal Lithiasis
Salmon: Multiple Myeloma